# Parasite Life Cycles

Dickson D. Despommier
John W. Karapelou

# Parasite Life Cycles

With 49 Life Cycle Drawings

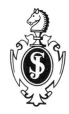

Springer-Verlag
New York Berlin Heidelberg
London Paris Tokyo

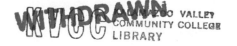

Dickson D. Despommier, Ph.D.
Professor of Public Health
  and of Microbiology
Division of Tropical Medicine
Columbia University
New York, N.Y. 10032, USA

John W. Karapelou
Chief Medical Illustrator
Center for Biomedical Communications
College of Physicians and Surgeons
Columbia University
New York, N.Y. 10032, USA

Library of Congress Cataloging-in-Publication Data
Despommier, Dickson D.
    Parasite life cycles / Dickson D. Despommier, John W. Karapelou.
        p.      cm.
    Bibliography: p.
    ISBN 0-387-96486-X
    1. Protozoa.    2. Helminths.    3. Parasites.    I. Karapelou, John W.
II. Title.
QL366.D47 1987

Typeset by Arcata Graphics/Kingsport, Kingsport, Tennessee.
Printed and bound by Arcata Graphics/Halliday, West Hanover, Massachusetts.
Printed in the United States of America

9 8 7 6 5 4 3 2 1

ISBN 0-387-96486-X Springer-Verlag New York Berlin Heidelberg
ISBN 3-540-96486-X Springer-Verlag Berlin Heidelberg New York

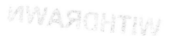

To Joan and Sam, and to
Nancy, John and Christina

# Acknowledgments

We thank Larry Carter for his vision and belief in this project from its inception. We thank Drs. Philip A. D'Alesandro, Suzanne Holmes Giannini, William C. Campbell, Bernard Fried, Larry Roberts, and Meredith Behr for reviewing various aspects of the book. We especially thank Drs. Harold W. Brown and Kathleen Hussey for amassing an outstanding collection of parasite material from which we derived much of what is illustrated throughout the book. We thank Mrs. Terri Terilli for pushing us when we had to be pushed and for encouraging us to continue. We also thank her for her skillful handling of the typing of the manuscript.

# Contents

## Part 3    Trematoda

## Part 4    Nematoda

# Introduction

The concept of parasitism has fascinated scientists for centuries, and over the last one hundred years, the field of parasitology has assumed its place as a full member of the ecological sciences. In the early days of parasitology research, the life cycles of these interesting organisms were the focal point of studies, thereby revealing the ways in which they complete their often complex journeys from one stage to the next.

A central theme has emerged from the now extensive life cycle literature; namely that each developmental stage is dependent upon environmental cues in order for it to progress to the next stage. Elucidation of the precise conditions needed to elicit stage-specific behavior has often taken years of laboratory and field work. Thus, we have come to appreciate the complexities of each parasite through these many efforts.

Life cycles of protozoan and helminthic parasites continue to hold the attention of a small but hearty group of biologists, so that our knowledge of parasite life styles continues to unfold.

Many species of parasitic protozoans and helminths occupy, sequentially, several microenvironments and invertebrate vectors during their development to reproductive adulthood. One need only review the life cycle of the fish tapeworm, *Diphyllobothrium latum,* in order to fully comprehend the term "complex" life cycle. The numerous sites selected by parasitic organisms infecting the human as the definitive host is reflected in the rich diversity of organisms that have evolved and prospered at our expense. In contrast, plasmodia, the causative agent of malaria, are actually parasites of the female anopheline mosquito, with the human serving as the intermediate host. In other cases, such as with trichinella, humans are but one of many species of mammalian hosts susceptible to infection.

In the text that follows, we have attempted to distill out and present the essentials of the life cycles of parasites that infect the human host without detracting from the complexities of them.

We decided that this is best done with a maximum of detailed illustrations and a minimum of words.

We have tried to depict each step of the process of infection in such a way that both the uninitiated and experienced biologist can gain insight into the host-parasite relationship. The selected reading list provided at the back of the text is intended to lead the interested reader to more complete biological information. Monographs on specific parasites are particularly useful, especially those written after 1980, and we have striven to list most of them.

The text, itself, is organized in such a way that the reader is introduced first to the general concepts of the major group (e.g., Protozoa, Nematoda, etc.). Next, the classification of each group is listed, at least as far down in the classification scheme as Family. In some cases, only Orders are listed, due to constraints of space. For classifications down to species, monographs dealing with each Family must be consulted. Most parasites in each phyla which infect the human host are presented pictorially, accompanied by a short text describing the essentials of their life cycle. Each illustration is a synthesis derived from information gathered from a wide variety of sources, including histopathological tissue sections, whole mounted material and gross specimens. Finally, the complete classification of each parasite depicted is given.

It is our hope that having the life cycles of all major protozoan and helminthic parasites that infect the human host illustrated in a single volume will stimulate interest in them among those not yet familiar with them, and serve as a ready source of information to those whose job it is to transmit the excitement of the field of parasitology to the rest of the scientific community.

Dickson D. Despommier
John W. Karapelou

# 1    Protozoa

# General Characteristics of the Protozoa

Approximately 66,000 species of protozoans have been described; about 10,000 of these are parasitic. Protozoans are single-celled organisms, exhibiting extensive diversity in all aspects of their biology. For example protozoans vary in their means of locomotion, and, to a great extent, this is the basis for their classification. They all exhibit some form of motility, often utilizing specialized organelles for that purpose (e.g., cilia and flagella). It is not known which motility mechanism(s) are employed by *Plasmodium* or the coccidae, since they do not possess any obvious locomotor organelles. Most species of protozoa are free-living and occupy niches as extreme as bottom sediments in deep marine trenches and geothermal springs. Similarly, parasitic protozoa show a wide variety of patterns for host selection and for site selection within a given host. Many are vectorborne—parasites in both cold-blooded and warm-blooded hosts. Literally every available niche within the human host can be parasitized.

All protozoa, be they free-living or parasitic, must carry out growth and replication within the confines of their unit membranes. Because of this, protozoans have been naturally selected for having uniquely solved various problems related to food-gathering and food-processing. Thus, their cytoplasm, depending upon the species, may contain highly specialized organelles that aid them in either aerobic or anaerobic energy metabolism.

Morphologically, protozoa vary in size from 1.5 µm to 50 mm in diameter. Division is accomplished by a wide variety of related mechanisms, with binary fission being the most common. Sexual reproduction also is a frequent reproductive strategy, and is particularly important for the coccidae and plasmodia. Protozoans parasitic for humans include representatives from 4 of the 7 groups, namely, Sarcomastigophora, Apicomplexa, Microspora, and Ciliophora. For brevity, and for relevance to the parasites in question, the classification presented here does not include suborder or family designations. However, the complete taxonomy for each parasite is given to aid readers when they consult the appropriate literature on a particular taxon.

# Classification

**Bold type** indicates orders represented in book by parasites

Kingdom: Protista
  Phylum: Sarcomastigophora
    Subphylum: Mastigophora
      Class: Phytomastigophorea
        Order: Cryptomonadida
        Order: Dinoflagellida
        Order: Euglenida
        Order: Chrysomonadida
        Order: Heterochlorida
        Order: Chloromonadida
        Order: Prymnesiida
        Order: Volvocida
        Order: Prasinomonadida
        Order: Silicoflagellida
      Class: Zoomastigophorea
        Order: Choanoflagellida
        **Order: Kinetoplastida**
        Order: Proteromonadida
        Order: Retortamonadida
        Order: Diplomonadida
        Order: Oxymonadida
      Superorder: Parabasalidea
        **Order: Trichomonadida**
        Order: Hypermastigida
    Subphylum: Opalinata
      Class: Opalinatea
        Order: Opalinida
    Subphylum: Sarcodina
      Superclass: Rhizopoda
      Class: Lobosea
        Subclass: Gymnamoebia
        **Order: Amoebida**
        Order: Schizopyrenida
        Order: Pelobiontida
        Subclass: Testacealobosia
        Order: Arcellinida
        Order: Trichosida
      Class: Acarpomyxea
        Order: Leptomyxida
        Order: Stereomyxida
      Class: Acrasea
        Order: Acrasida
      Class: Eumycetozoae
        Subclass: Protostelia
        Order: Protosteliida
        Subclass: Dictyosteliia
        Order: Dictyosteliida

        Subclass: Myxogastria
        Order: Echinosteliida
        Order: Liceida
        Order: Trichiida
        Order: Stemonitida
        Order: Physarida
      Class: Plasmodiophorea
        Order: Plasmodiophorida
      Class: Filosea
        Order: Aconchulinida
        Order: Gromiida
      Class: Granuloreticulosea
        Order: Athalamida
        Order: Monothalamida
        Order: Foraminiferida
      Class: Xenophyophorea
        Order: Psamminida
        Order: Stannomida
    Superclass: Actinopoda
      Class: Acantharea
        Order: Holacanthida
        Order: Symphyacanthida
        Order: Chaunacanthida
        Order: Arthracanthida
        Order: Actineliida
      Class: Polycystinea
        Order: Spumellarida
        Order: Nassellarida
      Class: Phaeodarea
        Order: Phaeocystida
        Order: Phaeosphaerida
        Order: Phaeocalpida
        Order: Phaeogromida
        Order: Phaeoconchida
        Order: Phaeodendrida
      Class: Heliozoea
        Order: Desmothoracida
        Order: Actinophryida
        Order: Taxopodida
        Order: Centrohelida
  Phylum: Labyrinthomorpha
    Class: Labyrinthulea
      Order: Labyrinthulida
  Phylum: Apicomplexa
    Class: Perkinsea
      Order: Perkinsida
    Class: Sporozoea

Subclass: Gregarinia
    Order: Archigregarinida
    Order: Eugregarinida
    Order: Neogregarinida
Subclass: Coccidia
    Order: Agamococcidiida
    Order: Protococcidiida
    **Order: Eucoccidiida**
Subclass: Piroplasmia
    Order: Piroplasmida
Phylum: Microspora
  Class: Rudimicrosporea
    Order: Metchnikovellida
  Class: Microsporea
    Order: Minisporida
    Order: Microsporida
Phylum: Ascetospora
  Class: Stellatosporea
    Order: Occlusosporida
    Order: Balanosporida
  Class: Paramyxea
    Order: Paramyxida
Phylum: Myxozoa
  Class: Myxosporea
    Order: Bivalvulida
    Order: Multivalvulida
  Class: Actinosporea
  Subclass: Actinomyxia
Phylum: Ciliophora
  Class: Kinetofragminophorea
  Subclass: Gymnostomatia
    Order: Prostomatida
    Order: Pleurostomatida

Order: Primociliatida
Order: Karyorelictida
Subclass: Vestibuliferia
    **Order: Trichostomatida**
Order: Entodiniomorphida
Order: Colpodida
Subclass: Hypostomatia
  Superorder: Nassulidea
    Order: Synhymeniida
    Order: Nassulida
  Superorder: Phyllopharyngidea
    Order: Crytophorida
    Order: Chonotrichida
  Superorder: Rhynchodea
    Order: Rhynchodida
  Superorder: Apostomatidea
    Order: Apostomatida
Subclass: Suctoria
    Order: Suctorida
Class: Oligohymenophorea
Subclass: Hymenostomatida
    Order: Hymenostomatida
    Order: Scuticociliatida
    Order: Astomatida
Subclass: Peritrichia
    Order: Peritrichida
Class: Polymenophorea
Subclass: Spirotrichia
    Order: Heterotrichida
    Order: Odontostomatida
    Order: Oligotrichida
    Order: Hypotrichida

# Trypanosoma Cruzi

1a  The infective stage of *Trypanosoma cruzi* is the metacyclic trypomastigote. It is 15 μm in length and possesses a single nucleus and flagellum. The flagellum is continuous with the undulating membrane, and originates at the kinetoplast, a large organized collection of extranuclear DNA.

1b  Transmission of *T. cruzi* from person to person occurs in many ways. The most frequent way is by the triatomid insect vector (the "kissing" bug). Many species of "kissing" bugs are vectors, the most common of which belong to the genera *Panstrongylus, Triatoma,* and *Rhodnius.* Infection occurs shortly after an infected bug takes a blood meal. During the feeding process, the insect defecates on the host's skin near the bite wound. Its feces contain the infective trypomastigotes.

2  When the bug leaves the site, the host experiences a mild itching sensation and rubs the trypomastigotes into the bite wound. If the bug bites on the face near the eye or mouth, then organisms can infect through mucous membranes. Other ways of acquiring *T. cruzi* include blood transfusions, transplacental infection and sexual intercourse.

3a  Trypomastigotes enter a wide variety of cells at the site of the bite wound and transform into amastigotes. The amastigote is 3-5 μm in diameter and does not possess an external flagellum. The intracellular amastigotes replicate by binary fission.

3b  The host becomes hypersensitive to the parasite as the result of the extensive cellular destruction at the site of initial infection.

4a  Some amastigotes transform into trypomastigotes within dying host cells. After being released into the peripheral blood, trypomastigotes infect other sites in the body.

4b  At this point in the infection any tissue may harbor parasites, including heart muscle (shown here) and nervous tissue (e.g., myenteric plexus). Transformation from amastigotes to trypomastigotes can occur at any site.

4c  The trypomastigotes penetrate new cells, transform to amastigotes, and begin the replication process again.

5  The triatomid bug becomes infected when it takes a blood meal from an individual containing trypomastigotes.

6  Trypomastigotes rapidly transform into dividing epimastigotes within the midgut of the bug, resulting in thousands of new parasites. Epimastigotes differentiate into metacyclic trypomastigotes within the hindgut. This is the infective stage of the parasite.

7  All mammals are susceptible to infection and can serve as reservoir hosts. The sloth, the oppossum, and various rodents, are important in maintaining the sylvatic cycle.

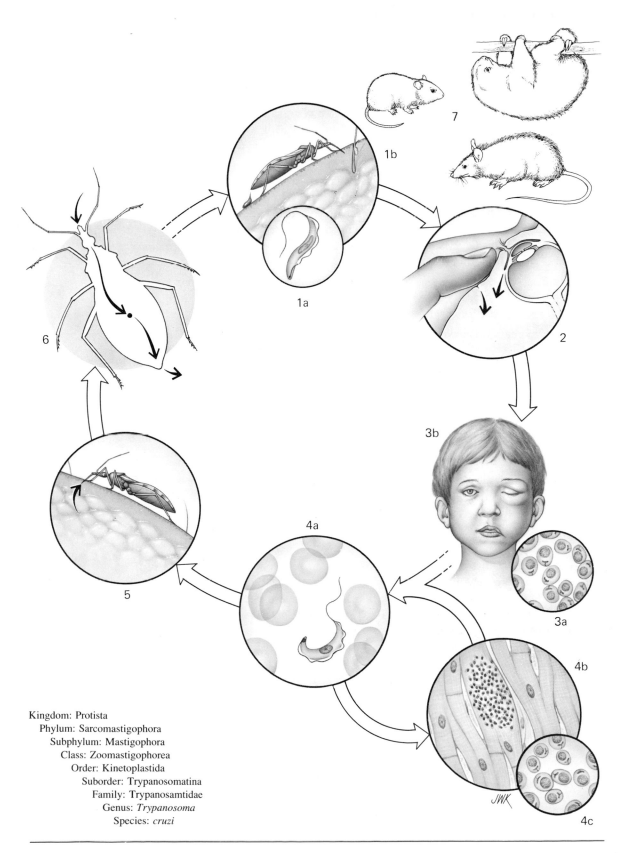

Kingdom: Protista
Phylum: Sarcomastigophora
Subphylum: Mastigophora
Class: Zoomastigophorea
Order: Kinetoplastida
Suborder: Trypanosomatina
Family: Trypanosamtidae
Genus: *Trypanosoma*
Species: *cruzi*

# Trypanosoma Brucei Gambiense

1a  The infective stage of *Trypanosoma brucei gambiense* is the metacyclic trypomastigote. This stage is about 12–15 μm in length, and it possesses a single nucleus and a flagellum. The flagellum is continuous with the undulating membrane and originates at the kinetoplast.

1b  Transmission of *T. b. gambiense* occurs when an infected tsetse fly takes a blood meal. The metacyclic trypomastigotes are injected into the bite wound along with the fly's salivary secretions. The metacyclic trypomastigote rapidly transforms into the bloodstream trypomastigote and begins to replicate by binary fission. Tsetse flies in the genus *Glossina* are capable of transmitting *T. b. gambiense; G. palpalis* and *G. tachinoides* are the most common ones.

2  A primary chancre develops at the site of the bite wound, with trypomastigotes being found extracellularly in various fluid spaces within it. This stage of the infection can last for several weeks to several months.

3  The trypomastigotes eventually find their way into the bloodstream and lymphatic system, where they continue to replicate by binary fission. They spend their entire life cycle extracellularly. The host responds to the infection by producing antibodies. The surface antigenic determinants are glycoproteins in the outer coat of the trypanosomes. The antibodies directed against them destroy, by agglutination and lysis, all antigenically identical organisms. A few trypanosomes with different surface antigens escape destruction. These variants multiply and replace those that were destroyed. The host again responds by producing antibodies against the new antigenic variant. In turn, a third variant arises. Thus yet another brood of trypanosomes takes over, the host responds once more, and this tug-of-war continues until the host is eventually overcome. Invasion of the central nervous system also occurs at this time, but is not part of the life cycle.

4  A tsetse fly becomes infected when it ingests a blood meal containing bloodstream trypomastigotes.

5  The bloodstream trypomastigotes transform into procyclic trypomastigotes in the midgut, where they then divide over a 10-day period, producing hundreds of new individuals. The procyclic trypomastigotes then leave the midgut for the salivary glands and transform into epimastigotes. More division occurs at this site, ultimately resulting in the production of thousands of metacyclic trypomastigotes, the infective stage for the human host. The entire process takes about 25–50 days to complete. Tsetse flies remain infective throughout their life. There are no known reservoir hosts for *T. b. gambiense*.

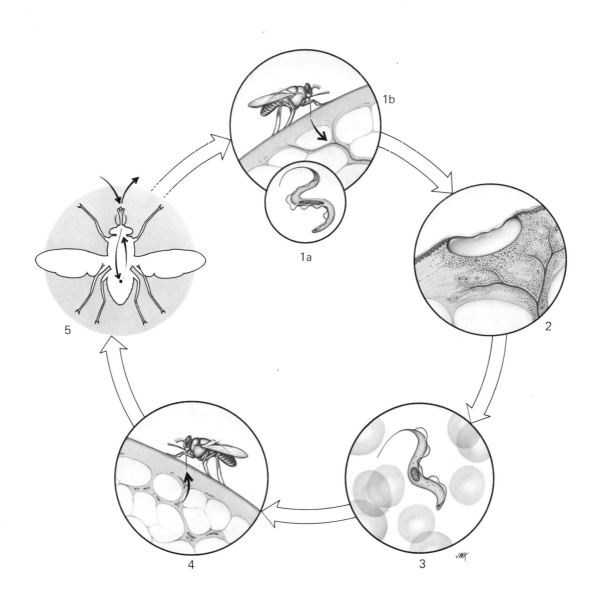

Kingdom: Protista
　Phylum: Sarcomastigophora
　　Subphylum: Mastigophora
　　　Class: Zoomastigophorea
　　　　Order: Kinetoplastida
　　　　　Suborder: Trypanosomatina
　　　　　　Genus: *Trypanosoma*
　　　　　　　Species: *brucei*
　　　　　　　　Subspecies: *rhodesiense*

# Trypanosoma Brucei Rhodesiense

1a  The life cycle of *Trypanosoma brucei rhodesiense* is similar to that of *T. b. gambiense*. The infective stage is the metacyclic trypomastigote, which lives within the salivary glands of the tsetse fly. This stage is approximately 15–20 μm in length, and it possesses a single nucleus, a flagellum attached to an undulating membrane, and a subterminal posterior kinetoplast.

1b  Infection occurs when an individual is bitten by an infected tsetse fly. The organisms are introduced into the skin of the host along with the salivary secretions of the infected insect. Important vectors of *T. b. rhodesiense* include *Glossina morsitans* and *G. pallidipes*.

2   The metacyclic trypomastigotes rapidly transform into bloodstream trypomastigotes within the extracellular spaces in the subcutaneous tissues. There, the parasites replicate by binary fission. A primary chancre is produced as the result of their presence.

3   The trypomastigotes eventually find their way into the bloodstream and the lymphatics, where they continue the replication cycle. Antigenic variation is a main feature of the life cycle of *T. b. rhodesiense*. Invasion of the cerebrospinal fluid of the central nervous system also occurs during this phase of the infection, but does not contribute to the life cycle.

4   The tsetse fly becomes infected when it ingests the trypomastigote while taking a blood meal from an infected individual.

5   The trypomastigote transforms within the lumen of the midgut into the procyclic trypomastigote. After several cycles of cell division, the procyclic trypomastigote migrates to the insect's salivary glands, where it differentiates further into the epimastigote and resumes division. Epimastigotes develop within the salivary gland into metacyclic trypomastigotes, the infective stage for the mammalian host.

6   Hartebeest and zebu cattle are important reservoir hosts for *T. b. rhodesiense*. Other mammals in East Africa also become infected with this parasite.

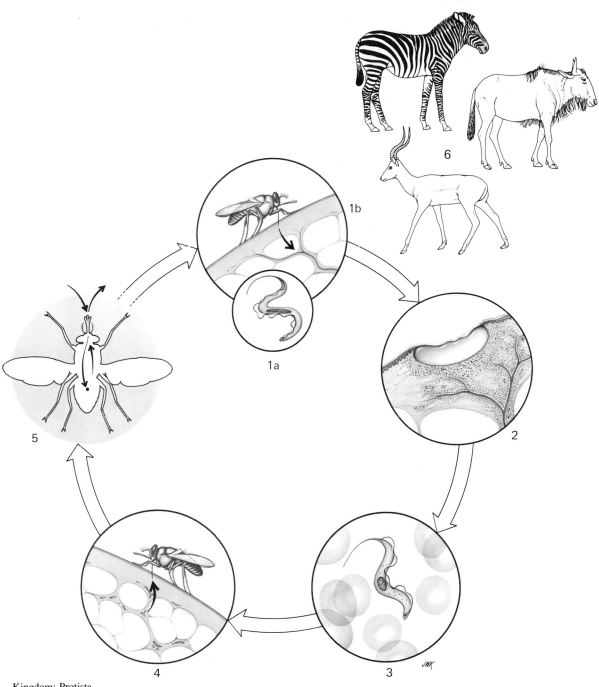

Kingdom: Protista
Phylum: Sarcomostigophora
Subphylum: Mastigophora
Class: Zoomastigophorea
Order: Kinetoplastida
Suborder: Trypanosomatina
Family: Trypanosamtidae
Genus: *Trypansoma*
Species: *brucei*
Subspecies: *gambiense*

# Leishmania Tropica and L. Mexicana

1a  The infective stage of *Leishmania tropica* and *L. mexicana* is the promastigote. This form of the organism lives in the midgut and mouthparts of the infected sand fly. It possesses a single nucleus, a flagellum, and a prominent subterminal anterior kinetoplast.

1b  *L. tropica* and *L. mexicana* are transmitted from person to person by the bite of an infected sand fly. Sand flies in the genus *Phlebotimus* are the most common vectors in Europe, the Middle East, and Asia, whereas *Lutzomyia* commonly transmits *L. mexicana* throughout Central and South America.

2a  Once the promastigote is injected into the skin, it is phagocytosed by a macrophage and rapidly transforms to the amastigote stage. Infection is limited to the cutaneous and subcutaneous tissues near the original site of infection.

2b  The amastigotes replicate within each macrophage by binary fission. Lysis of the host cell ensues.

2c  The reproductive cycle is repeated many times in the skin.

3a,b  Amastigotes within macrophages are ingested by sand flies when they take a blood meal from the infected margin of the ulcer.

4  Once inside the sand fly midgut, the amastigotes are freed from infected host cells by digestion. The parasites then transform into promastigotes, the infective stage for the mammalian host. Promastigotes undergo several cycles of division, then migrate to the proboscis where they await the taking of another blood meal.

5  *L. tropica* and *L. mexicana* can infect other animals, as well as man, with rodents and dogs serving as important reservoir hosts for both species.

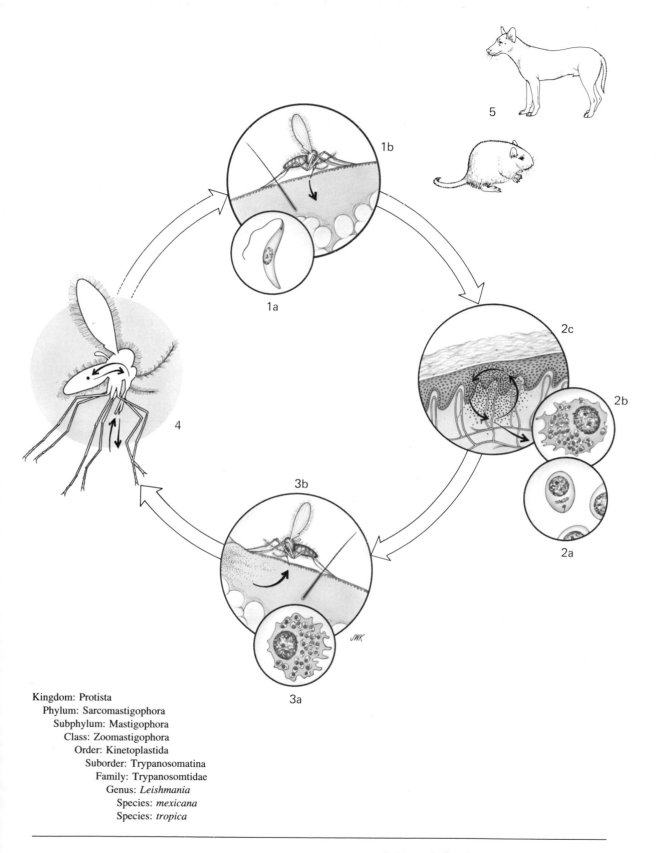

1b

1a

2c

2b

2a

3b

3a

JWK

4

5

Kingdom: Protista
Phylum: Sarcomastigophora
Subphylum: Mastigophora
Class: Zoomastigophora
Order: Kinetoplastida
Suborder: Trypanosomatina
Family: Trypanosomtidae
Genus: *Leishmania*
Species: *mexicana*
Species: *tropica*

# Leishmania Braziliensis

1a  The infective stage of *Leishmania braziliensis* is the promastigote. Promastigotes are 10–15 µm in length, and they possess a single nucleus, a flagellum, and a subterminal anterior kinetoplast. Sand flies in the genus *Lutzomyia* are the vectors of this parasite.

1b  Infection occurs when an infected sand fly takes a second blood meal. The parasites enter the bite wound with the salivary secretion.

2a  The promastigotes round up and lose their flagellum, becoming amastigotes.

2b  Transformation from promastigote to amastigote occurs within the parasitophorous vacuoles of macrophages shortly after the phagocytes ingest the parasites.

2c  The entire infection is limited to the subcutaneous tissue, with the growth and division of the parasites resulting in the death of the macrophages.

3a  The infected macrophages continue to die, releasing more amastigotes.

3b  Increased infection in the subcutaneous tissue near the bite wound leads to destruction of tissue, resulting in a craterform ulcer. Organisms are found at the edge of the lesion in living tissue.

3c  Infected macrophages can travel via the bloodstream to other parts of the body before dying and releasing their parasites. However, only macrophages at mucocutaneous junctions are susceptible to infection. Such metastases can lead to erosion of the soft palate.

3d  Infection at the mucocutaneous junction of the urogenital and anal regions can also occur.

4a  Infected macrophages at the margins of ulcers at any infection site can serve as the source of infection for sand flies.

4b  Sand flies acquire their infection during the taking of a blood meal.

5  Within the sand fly, the infected macrophages are digested in the midgut of the insect, liberating the amastigotes. The parasites rapidly transform into promastigotes, the infective stage for the mammalian host. After many replication cycles in the midgut, the promastigotes migrate into the proboscis of the insect and await the taking of another blood meal by the sand fly.

6  There are many reservoir hosts, including the sloth and several varieties of rodents.

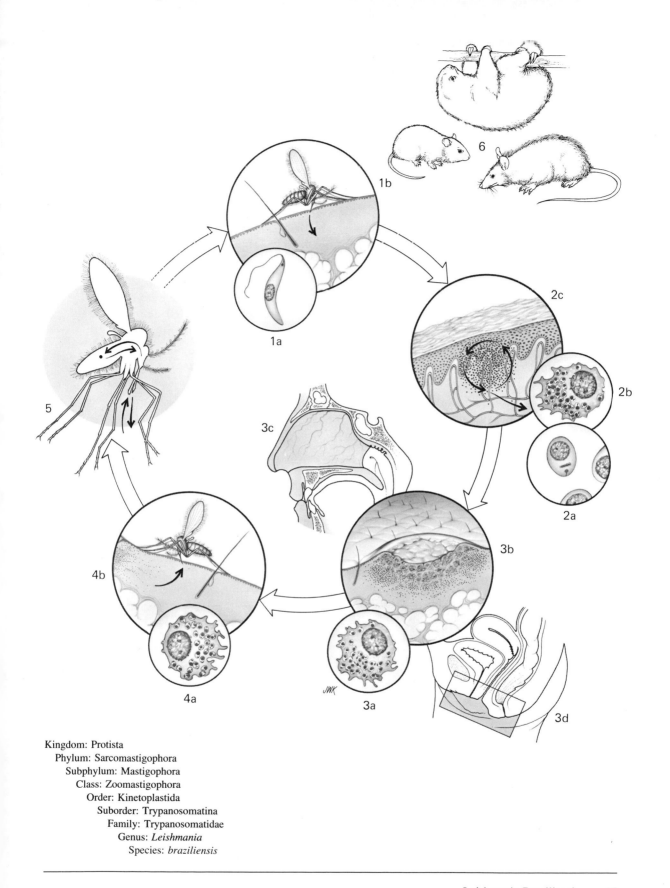

Kingdom: Protista
Phylum: Sarcomastigophora
Subphylum: Mastigophora
Class: Zoomastigophora
Order: Kinetoplastida
Suborder: Trypanosomatina
Family: Trypanosomatidae
Genus: *Leishmania*
Species: *braziliensis*

# Leishmania Donovani

1a  The promastigote is the infective stage for humans. It lives within the lumen of the proboscis of its vector, the sand fly.

1b  The infected sand fly transmits *L. donovani* from person to person by injecting the promastigotes into the skin of the mammalian host, along with salivary secretions, during the taking of a blood meal. Sand flies in the genus *Phlebotomus* are common vectors in Africa, the Middle East, and Asia, while *Lutzomyia* transmits *L. donovani* in Central and South America.

2a  The promastigotes are rapidly phagocytosed in the skin by macrophages.

2b  The promastigotes then transform to amastigotes. In contrast to *L. tropica, L. mexicana,* or *L. braziliensis,* the amastigotes are not restricted to skin, but are carried throughout the viscera, where they infect a wide variety of fixed and wandering macrophages.

3a-3c  Subsequent replication and host cell death results in widespread distribution of the infection within the reticuloendothelial system (e.g., spleen, 3a; bone marrow 3b; and liver 3c).

4  The sand fly acquires its infection by ingesting an infected macrophage during the taking of a blood meal. Infected macrophages can be ingested from any bite wound site on the body, since infected cells are present throughout the peripheral circulation.

5  The amastigote transforms into the promastigote in the midgut of the sand fly. The parasites undergo several division cycles before migrating into the lumen of the proboscis, thereby completing the life cycle.

6  Many reservoir hosts exist in nature, the most important of which are the dog and the gerbil.

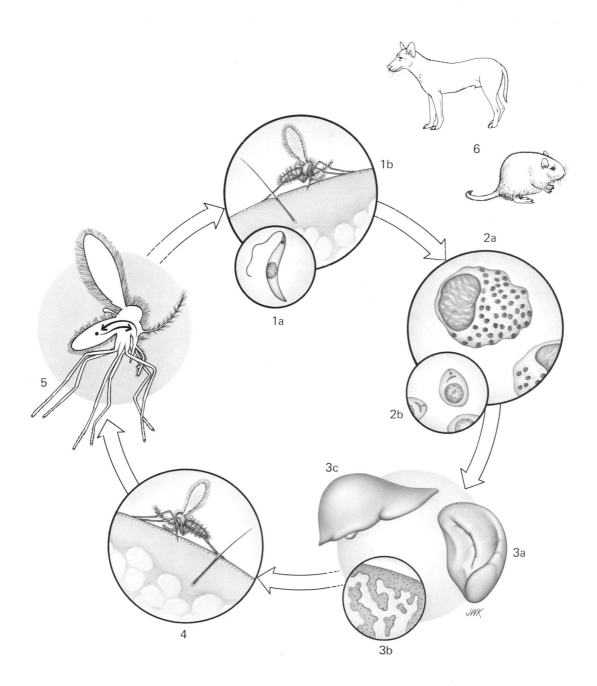

Kingdom: Protista
Phylum: Sarcomastigophora
Subphylum: Mastigophora
Class: Zoomastigophorea
Order: Kinetoplastida
Suborder: Trypanosomatina
Family: Trypanosomatidae
Genus: *Leishmania*
Species: *donovani*

# Giardia Lamblia

1a  The infective stage of *Giardia lamblia* is the cyst, which is approximately 15 μm long by 5 μm wide, and possesses four nuclei.

1b  The cyst must be ingested in feces-contaminated food or water for the life cycle to begin.

2   Excystment occurs in the small intestine, with a single cyst giving rise to two trophozoites. Each trophozoite is about 10–20 μm long by 7–10 μm wide and possesses six flagella.

3   The trophozoites live upon the surface of the villi in the small intestine.

4   *G. lamblia* adheres to the columnar cells by means of a disklike depression on its ventral surface, which functions as a sucker. Encystment occurs in the lumen of the small intestine, resulting in the production of infectious quadrinucleate cysts.

5   The cysts pass into the environment with the fecal mass where they can survive for extended periods of time.

6   Both dogs and beavers have been identified as important reservoir hosts for *G. lamblia,* although other mammals, such as deer, can also become infected.

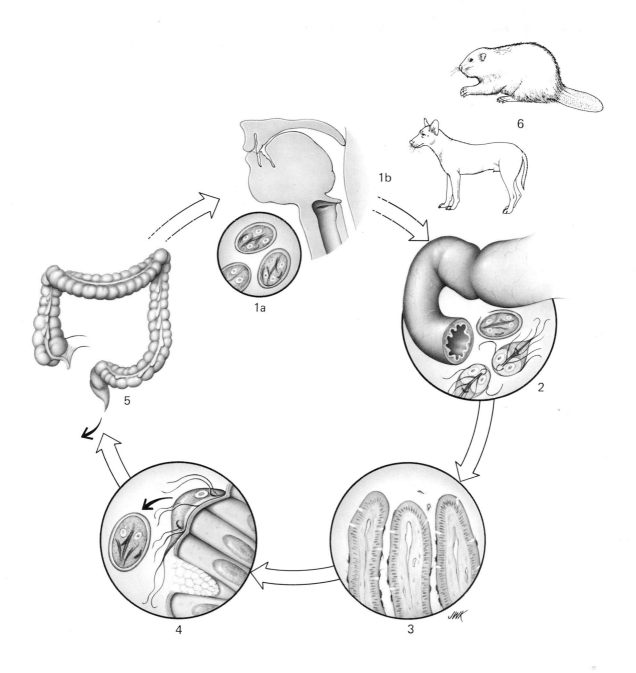

1a

1b

2

3

4

5

6

Kingdom: Protista
Phylum: Sarcomastigophora
Subphylum: Mastigophora
Class: Zoomastigophorea
Order: Diplomonadida
Suborder: Diplomonadina
Family: Hexamitidae
Genus: *Giardia*
Species: *lamblia*

# Trichomonas Vaginalis

1a  There is only one stage of *Trichomonas vaginalis,* namely, the trophozoite. It measures approximately 10–25 μm in diameter. *T. vaginalis* possesses a single undulating membrane and four flagella. In addition, its cytoplasm contains various subcellular particles, one of which, the hydrogenosome, plays an important role in anaerobic metabolism. *T. vaginalis* lives on the surface of the epithelium of the urogenital tract where it derives its energy through anaerobic metabolic pathways, secreting molecular hydrogen as one of its waste products.

1b  *T. vaginalis* is transmitted from person to person most commonly by sexual intercourse. Infection of the newborn female can occur by passage through the infected birth canal of the mother. In such cases, infections remain quiescent until puberty. There are no reservoir hosts for this infection.

2  In the male, the most commonly infected site is the epithelium of the urethra in the region of the prostate gland. The prostate gland itself may also harbor organisms.

3  Adults become infected during sexual intercourse with an infected partner.

4  Trophozoites only infect the surface epithelium of the vaginal tract and cervix in the female. They never invade the surface of the uterus or fallopian tubes. Trophozoites reproduce by binary fission.

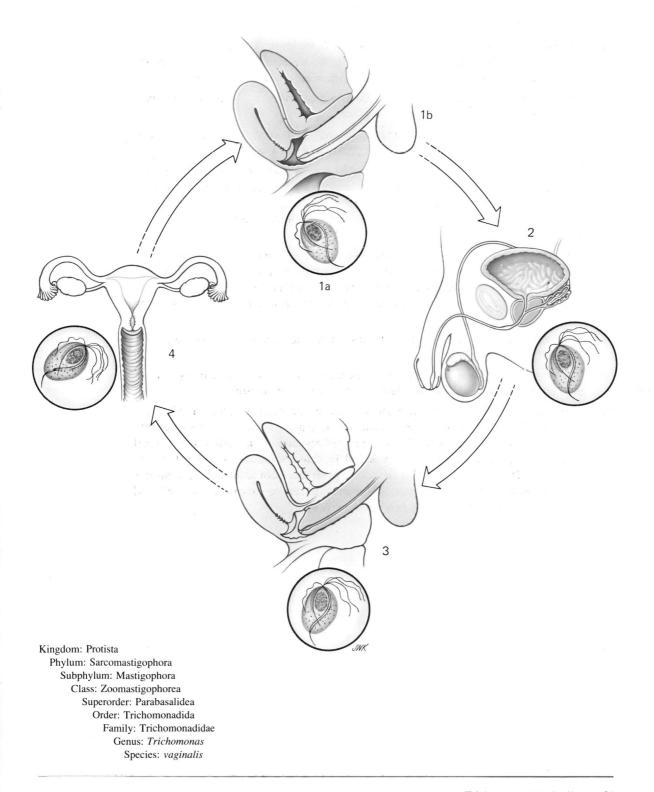

Kingdom: Protista
Phylum: Sarcomastigophora
Subphylum: Mastigophora
Class: Zoomastigophorea
Superorder: Parabasalidea
Order: Trichomonadida
Family: Trichomonadidae
Genus: *Trichomonas*
Species: *vaginalis*

# Entamoeba Histolytica

1a  The infective stage of *Entamoeba histolytica* is the cyst. The nonmotile cyst is 10–15 μm in diameter and contains four nuclei, each of which has a centrally located karyosome. It is surrounded by a resistant outer wall.

1b  The cyst must be swallowed in order for the life cycle to begin. Cysts are commonly ingested in feces-contaminated food or water.

2  Excystment occurs in the small intestine, during which time each nucleus divides once. Thus eight motile trophozoites are produced from a single cyst.

3a  The trophozoite varies in size from 20 to 30 μm in diameter. Its single nucleus contains a centrally located karyosome surrounded by even-sized and spaced chromatin at its periphery. The nucleus thus assumes the pattern of a bullseye. Ingested red cells may also be present in food vacuoles throughout the cytoplasm of *E. histolytica.*

3b  The trophozoites of *E. histolytica* live in the tissues of the large intestine where they feed on living cells and replicate by binary fission. The trophozoites can also take up residence in other organs, but in this case are unable to participate in the completion of the life cycle, since they cannot return to the lumen of the large intestine.

4a  Encystment occurs in the lumen of the large intestine. The trophozoite begins the process by "rounding up."

4b  The early cyst is characterized by the presence of the cyst wall, one or two nuclei and smoothe ended chromatoidal bars (ordered arrays of ribosomes).

4c  Cyst formation is complete when all four nuclei are present. Chromatoidal bars are usually not present in the cytoplasm of the mature cyst. Cysts pass out into the environment with the fecal mass and are resistant to a variety of physical conditions. In addition, they are not killed by dilute solutions of many types of chemicals. Therefore, they are able to survive in the feces-contaminated environment up to 1 month. While many species of mammals can be experimentally infected with *E. histolytica,* none serves as a reservoir host.

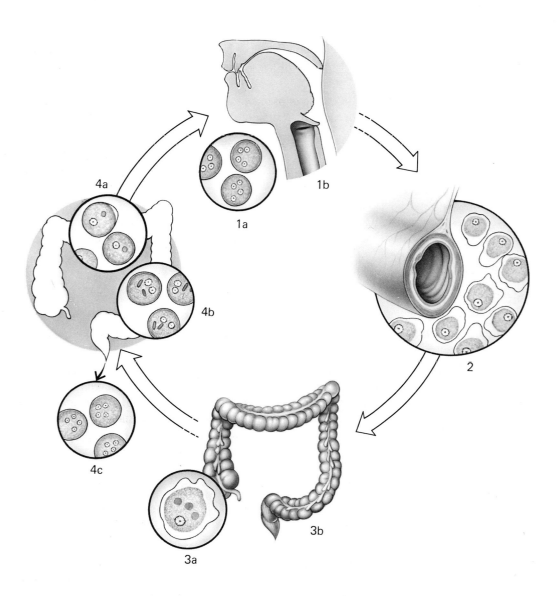

1a

1b

4a

4b

4c

2

3a

3b

Kingdom: Protista
Phylum: Sarcomastigophora
Subphylum: Sarcodina
Superclass: Rhizopoda
Class: Lobosea
Subclass: Gymnamoebia
Order: Amoebida
Suborder: Tubulina
Family: Entamoebidae
Genus: *Entamoeba*
Species: *histolytica*

# Toxoplasma Gondii

## Asexual cycle

1a  The infective stage of *T. gondii* for the human host is the pseudocyst. The pseudocyst is 30 μm to 100 μm in diameter, and contains hundreds to thousands of infectious units termed bradyzoites. *T. gondii* is an obligate intracellular parasite.

1b  Infection is frequently initiated by ingestion of pseudocysts contained in raw or undercooked unfrozen meats. In addition, infection can occur by ingestion of oocysts (5d) in the feces of cats experiencing active intestinal infection.

2a  The wall of either the pseudocyst or oocyst is broken down in the small intestine by host digestive enzymes releasing the bradyzoites or sporozoites, respectively, that then penetrate the columnar epithelium.

2b  It is probable that bradyzoites or sporozoites reach the liver by the hematogenous route where they are ingested by Küpffer cells. Once inside a cell, the organisms are referred to as tachyzoites. Liver parenchymal cells also become infected. Replication immediately follows entry into host cells.

3a  Macrophages transport *T. gondii* throughout the body. *T. gondii* survives and replicates within the macrophage parasitophorous vacuole by preventing the fusion of lysosomes with it.

3b  Division is by endodyogeny, a process of internal budding.

3c  The division cycle produces rosettes of organisms termed tachyzoites.

3d  Replication results in the lysis of the host cell. Organisms are phagocytosed by new macrophages or other cell types and repeat the cycle.

3e  Host resistance develops, slowing down the rate of reproduction of *T. gondii*, resulting in the pseudocyst. Replication occurs slowly within the pseudocyst, producing hundreds to thousands of bradyzoites. Pseudocysts can remain dormant within host tissues for years. Excystment occurs within the same host if cellular-based defense mechanisms are suppressed or significantly reduced.

4  The developing fetus can become infected via the placenta from the infected mother.

## Sexual Cycle

5a  The sexual cycle of *T. gondii* occurs only in feline hosts. The intermediate host (e.g., mouse) becomes infected by ingesting either oocysts or pseudocysts.

5b  The mouse develops pseudocysts throughout its own tissues.

5c  The cat becomes infected when it eats infected meat (e.g., rodent tissues) containing the pseudocysts or ingests oocysts. Bradyzoites or sporozoites penetrate columnar epithelial cells and differentiate into merozoites. Following replication, merozoites rupture infected epithelial cells and infect adjacent ones. Some merozoites differentiate into pre-sex cells termed macrogametocytes (♀) and microgametocytes (♂).

5d  The microgametocytes fuse with macrogametocytes, forming zygotes termed oocysts. Oocysts enter the lumen of the small intestine and are defecated. Each oocyst sporulates in the soil, producing eight infectious sporozoites, the infectious stage for the intermediate host. The asexual cycle can also occur in feline hosts.

6  *Toxoplasma gondii* can infect any mammal and all cell types within a given individual. No other parasite, be it virus, bacteria, fungus or helminth can match *T. gondii* for its diversity of host range or its lack of site specificity within the host.

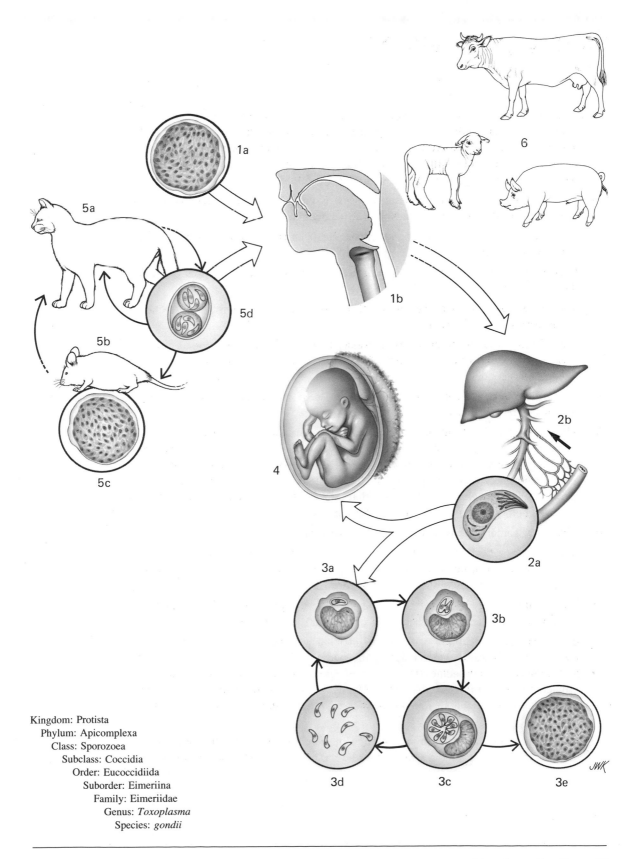

Kingdom: Protista
Phylum: Apicomplexa
Class: Sporozoea
Subclass: Coccidia
Order: Eucoccidiida
Suborder: Eimeriina
Family: Eimeriidae
Genus: *Toxoplasma*
Species: *gondii*

# Cryptosporidium Sp.

1a  The sporulated oocyst is the infectious stage of *Cryptosporidium* sp. Each oocyst measures 3–5 μm in diameter, and contains four infectious units termed sporozoites and a characteristic refractile residual body. It is not known whether or not there is more than one species of *Cryptosporidium,* since the organism is morphologically indistinguishable regardless of the source of infection.

1b  Infection begins when the sporulated oocyst is ingested. Feces-contaminated food and water are the most common sources of infection.

2   The oocyst releases the sporozoites in the small intestine upon contact with host digestive enzymes.

3a  Each sporozoite is capable of infecting a columnar epithelial cell, thus beginning the asexual cycle.

3b  The sporozoite attaches to the surface of the epithelial cell and embeds itself down to the base of the microvilli.

3c  The parasite induces the host cell to extend the microvilli up and around its entire surface, following which the parasite differentiates into the trophozoite. The parasite is now intracellular.

3d  The trophozoite transforms into the schizont, resulting in the production of eight organisms termed merozoites.

3e  The merozoites burst out of their membrane-bound host cell and are now capable of infecting another epithelial cell. This cycle usually occurs once more, now resulting in the production of only four merozoites. However, in individuals suffering from immunodeficiencies, such as AIDS, the merozoites can reinfect for many cycles. Alternatively, a newly arrived merozoite may differentiate into either a microgametocyte (♂) or a macrogametocyte (♀).

4a  The microgametocyte produces 12 to 16 microgametes.

4b  The microgametes burst out of their infected host cell. Each microgamete is able to fuse with a macrogametocyte (shown on left). The macrogametocyte remains within the host cell cytoplasm until it is fertilized.

5   The resulting zygote, termed the oocyst, differentiates, secretes an impervious outer wall, and then enters the lumen of the small intestine.

6   Before leaving the lumen of the large intestine with the fecal mass, the fertilized oocyst is unsporulated. Upon reaching the external environment, the oocyst immediately sporulates, thus achieving infectivity. Sporulation can also occur if the unsporulated oocyst is ingested. The entire life cycle takes approximately 2 to 4 weeks in healthy individuals. In immunosuppressed persons, the cycle can go on indefinitely.

7   *Cryptosporidium* can initiate infection in a wide variety of mammalian species. Calves and suckling pigs are thought to be the most common reservoir hosts.

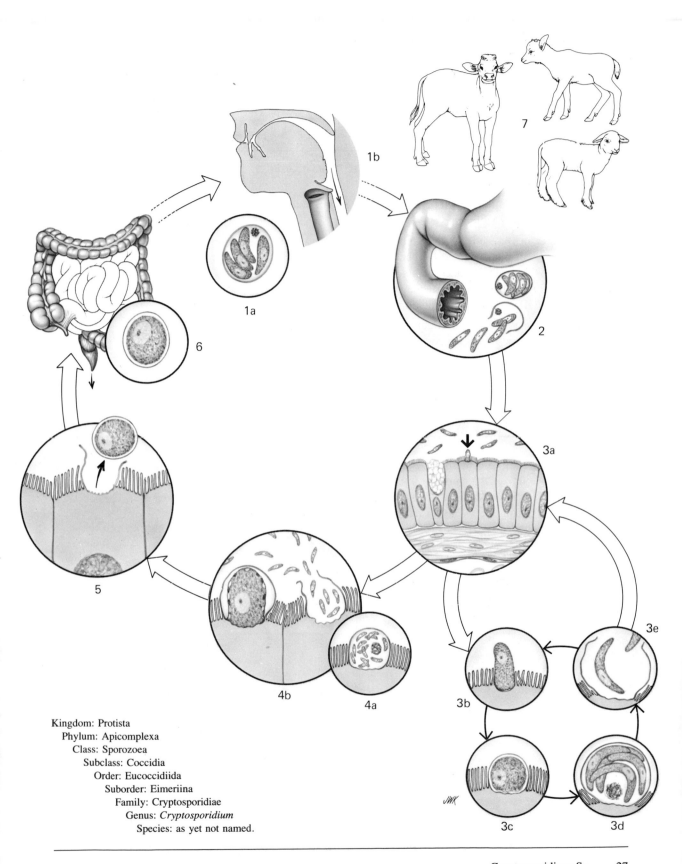

Kingdom: Protista
Phylum: Apicomplexa
Class: Sporozoea
Subclass: Coccidia
Order: Eucoccidiida
Suborder: Eimeriina
Family: Cryptosporidiae
Genus: *Cryptosporidium*
Species: as yet not named.

# Plasmodium Vivax

## Sexual Cycle (Mosquito)

1 Different species of anopheline mosquitoes transmit different species of malaria. The mosquito becomes infected when she ingests the macrogametocytes (♀) and microgametocytes (♂) present in the peripheral blood of an infected human (intermediate host).

2 The red cell cytoplasm is digested away from the gametocytes within the lumen of the mosquito's stomach.

3 Microgametocytes differentiate and divide into 6 to 8 flagellated microgametes. The process of microgamete formation is termed exflagellation. Each microgamete can fuse with a single macrogamete, thus forming a zygote termed the ookinete. After fusion of the two nuclei, the organism becomes diploid. Ookinete formation takes about 18 hours for completion.

4 The ookinete penetrates between the columnar epithelium and comes to rest just under the connective tissue sheath and further differentiates into the oocyst.

5 Each oocyst undergoes nuclear reduction, then a series of nuclear and cytoplasmic division cycles, resulting in the production of thousands of haploid sporozoites. Sporozoite production is complete within 8–10 days after ingestion of gametocytes. The sporozoites enter the hemocoel by penetrating the wall of the oocyst.

6a Each sporozoite is approximately 2–3 μm long and possesses a single centrally located nucleus.

6b Sporozoites site select within the cytoplasm of the cuboidal epithelium lining the salivary glands and the lumen of the glands themselves. They gain entrance into the human intermediate host when the mosquito injects them, together with salivary secretions, during the taking of her next blood meal.

7 Female mosquitoes in the genus *Anopheles* are the definitive hosts for all species of malaria, including *Plasmodium vixax*.

Note: The same general scheme of sexual development (*1–6b*) applies to *P. ovale, P. falciparum,* and *P. malariae,* as well, although the exact timing for each stage of development varies from species to species.

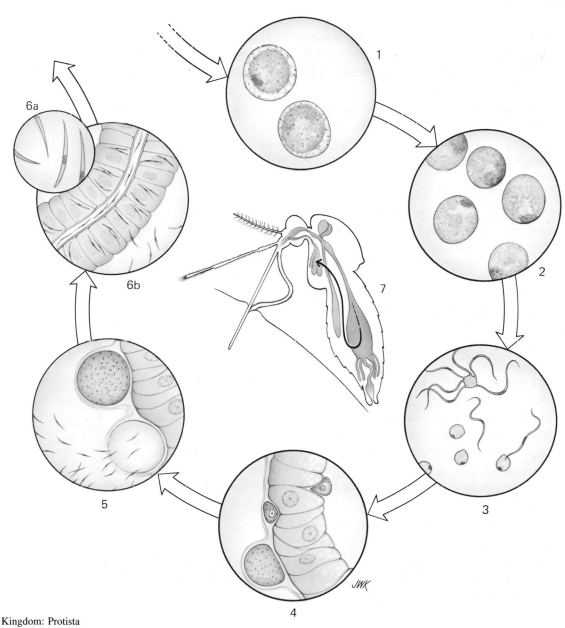

6a

6b

1

2

3

4

5

7

Kingdom: Protista
Phylum: Apicomplexa
Class: Sporozoea
Subclass: Coccidia
Order: Eucoccidiida
Suborder: Haemosporina
Family: Plasmodiidae
Genus: *Plasmodium*
Species: *vivax*

# Plasmodium Vivax

## Asexual Cycle

1a  The sporozoite is the infectious stage and is 2–3 μm long.

1b  Sporozoites are injected, along with the salivary secretion of the mosquito, into the human intermediate host when an infected female anopheline mosquito takes a second or third blood meal.

2a  The sporozoites travel via the hematogenous route to the liver, where they enter parenchymal cells, thereby initiating the exoerythrocytic cycle.

2b  Following differentiation into merozoites, the organisms divide by schizogony into hundreds of infectious units.

3   The exoerythrocytic cycle takes about 6–8 days to complete, culminating in the rupture of the infected parenchymal cell, with the consequent release of about 10,000 parasites into the bloodstream. Merozoites cannot enter new parenchymal cells but can enter red blood cells. Entry into the red cell signals the onset of the erythrocytic cycle. Some merozoites, instead of repeatedly dividing within the parenchymal cell, differentiate into a dormant non-dividing stage termed a hypnozoite (*). This stage can go on to replicate into merozoites at a later time in the infection. Activation of hypnozoites results in a relapse of infection and can occur at any time after initial infection up to 5 years.

4a  Replication of *P. vivax* within the red blood cell occurs through an asexual division process, and begins with the trophozoite stage.

4b  The single nucleated trophozoite grows within the red cell, feeding mainly upon the protein portion of hemoglobin. During this time, the infected red cell becomes deformed and enlarged.

4c  Nuclear division occurs repeatedly, resulting in 16 to 32 nuclei. The cytoplasm then divides, separating each nucleus into a merozoite.

4d  The infected red cell ruptures, releasing the parasites into the bloodstream. After entering a new red cell, the division cycle is repeated. One erythrocytic cycle is completed within 41–45 hours. Some early trophozoites (4a), instead of dividing, differentiate into presexual stages.

5a  The macrogametocyte is the female presexual stage

5b  The microgametocyte is the male presexual stage.

5c  These two stages are infective for the definitive host, the female anopheline mosquito, and are acquired by the insect when she takes a blood meal. There are no reservoir hosts for any species of human malaria.

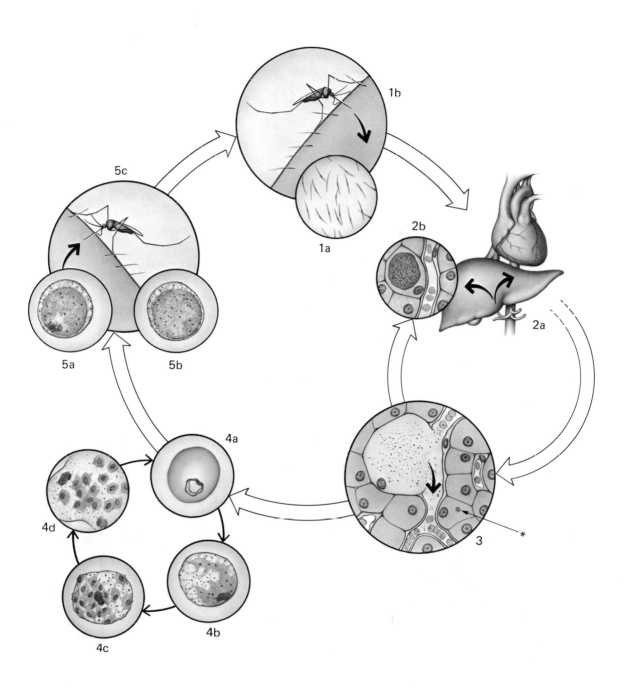

# Plasmodium Ovale

## Asexual Cycle

1a  The sporozoite is the infectious stage and is 2–3 μm long.

1b  The sporozoites of *Plasmodium ovale* are injected, along with the salivary secretions of the mosquito, into the host when an infected female anopheline mosquito takes a second or third blood meal.

2a  Sporozoites are passively carried by the bloodstream to all organs, but only survive if they reach the liver. In the liver, the sporozoites break out of the capillaries and penetrate parenchymal cells, initiating the exoerythrocytic cycle.

2b  The parasites differentiate into merozoites. Some merozoites differentiate further into hypnozoites (*), a nondividing stage, while others undergo multiple divisions, resulting in the formation of mature schizonts. Each schizont gives rise to about 15,000 organisms and takes 9 days to fully mature.

3  Mature schizonts rupture, thereby releasing merozoites into adjacent capillaries. Invasion of red cells by the merozoites then ensues, thus beginning the erythrocytic cycle. Merozoites are unable to invade parenchymal cells. Hypnozoites can mature into schizonts with attendant release of merozoites, thus initiating a new erythrocytic cycle. When this occurs, the infected individual experiences a relapse of the infection. Relapses can apparently occur at anytime up to 5 years after the initial infection.

4a  Invasion of a red cell by a merozoite results in the development of the early trophozoite stage, known as the signet ring stage.

4b  Growth of the trophozoite culminates in the digestion of most of the hemoglobin of the red cell. A particular waste product of hemoglobin digestion, hemozoin, accumulates in the unoccupied portion of host cell cytoplasm. The overall diameter of the infected red cell increases and its shape becomes irregular.

4c  Nuclear division takes place within a syncytium of parasite cytoplasm. Following nuclear division, the cytoplasm divides. Thus 8 to 10 merozoites are formed and are collectively termed the mature schizont. The entire process of nuclear and cytoplasmic division is termed schizogony.

4d  The mature schizont ruptures, freeing its complement of merozoites into the bloodstream. Each released merozoite has the opportunity to invade a new red cell. The erythrocytic cycle takes 49–50 hours to complete. Not all merozoites that enter red cells divide. Rather, some differentiate into pre-sex cells.

5a  The female pre-sex cell is termed the macrogametocyte.

5b  The male pre-sex cell is called the microgametocyte.

5c  The mosquito acquires her infection by ingesting macro and microgametocytes along with her blood meal. There are no reservoir hosts for any species of human malaria.

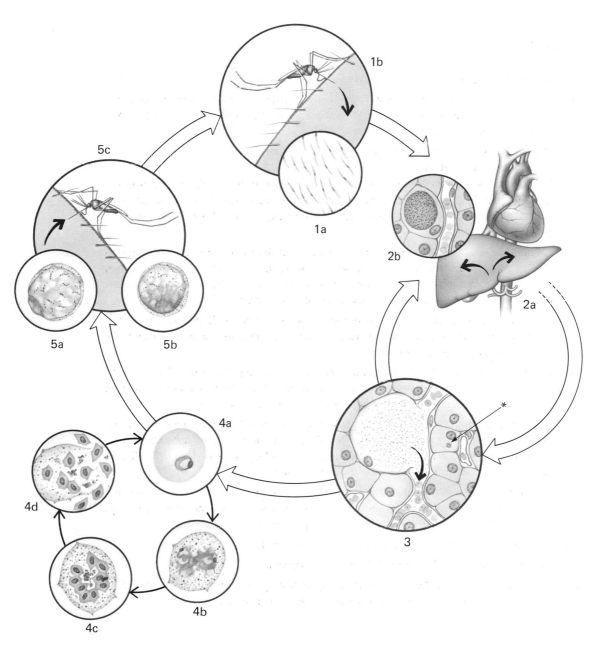

1a
1b
2a
2b
3
*
4a
4b
4c
4d
5a
5b
5c

Kingdom: Protista
Phylum: Apicomplexa
Class: Sporozoea
Subclass: Coccidia
Order: Eucoccidiida
Suborder: Haemosporina
Family: Plasmodiidae
Genus: *Plasmodium*
Species: *ovale*

# Plasmodium Malariae

## Asexual Cycle

1a  The sporozoite is 2–3 μm long and is the infectious stage.

1b  Infection in the human host by *Plasmodium malariae* begins when the sporozoites are injected, along with the salivary secretion, into the blood vessels in the skin by an infected female anopheline mosquito.

2a  The sporozoites are passively carried to the liver as well as to other parts of the body by the bloodstream.

2b  In the liver, the sporozoites enter parenchymal cells and differentiate into merozoites, signaling the beginning of the exoerythrocytic cycle. Division of the merozoites results in the production of about 2,000 parasites, taking about 12–16 days to complete.

3   The mature schizont ruptures the infected cell and the merozoites enter the bloodstream. Merozoites are unable to invade parenchymal cells. *P. malariae* does not form hypnozoites, therefore it is not a cause of relapsing malaria. However, initial infections can last for up to 30 years, even after treatment.

4a  The erythrocytic cycle starts with the invasion of the red cell by the merozoite. As with all other species of malaria, the early trophozoite stage is commonly referred to as the signet ring stage.

4b  The trophozoite feeds upon the protein portion of hemoglobin and enlarges to fill most of the host cell cytoplasm. Unlike *P. vivax* and *P. ovale*, *P. malariae* infection does not alter either the size or shape of the infected erythrocyte.

4c  Nuclear and cytoplasmic division (schizogony) sequentially occur, resulting in the production of merozoites. Hemozoin, a solid waste product of hemoglobin digestion, is sequestered into the center of the infected red cell cytoplasm. The red cell plus the organisms inside it is called the mature schizont.

4d  The infected red cell ruptures, thereby releasing the parasites. Invasion of another red cell by a merozoite initiates another cycle of division. Some merozoites, instead of undergoing schizogony, differentiate into pre-sex cells.

5a  The female pre-sex cell is called the macrogametocyte.

5b  The male pre-sex cell is termed the microgametocyte.

5c  The female mosquito becomes infected by ingesting both types of pre-sex cells. There are no reservoir hosts for any species of human malaria.

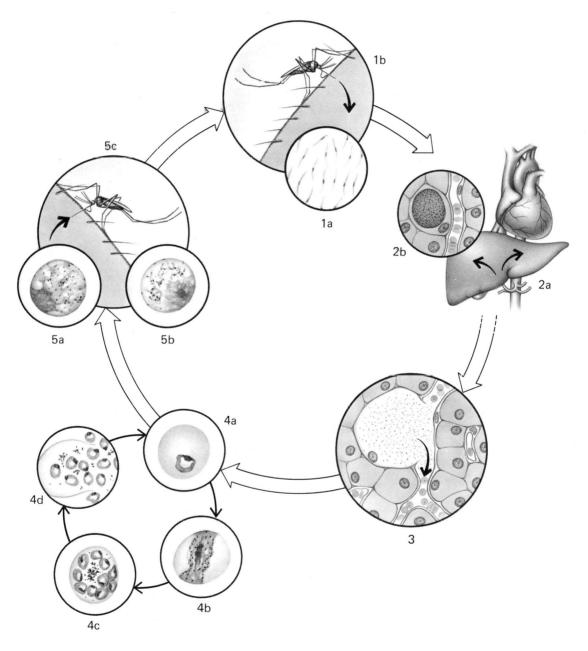

Kingdom: Protista
  Phylum: Apicomplexa
    Class: Sporozoea
      Subclass: Coccidia
        Order: Eucoccidiida
          Suborder: Haemosporina
            Family: Plasmodiidae
              Genus: *Plasmodium*
                Species: *malariae*

# Plasmodium Falciparum

## Asexual Cycle

1a  The sporozoite is the infectious stage and is 2–3 μm in length.

1b  Infection begins in the human host when an infected female anopheline mosquito injects sporozoites, along with the salivary secretion, into blood vessels in the skin while she is taking a second or third blood meal.

2a  The bloodstream transports the sporozoites to all parts of the body. However, in order to continue the life cycle, sporozoites must reach the liver and penetrate into parenchymal cells.

2b  Once in their intracellular niche, each sporozoite differentiates into a merozoite and begins to divide, beginning the exoerythrocytic cycle. Schizogony takes 5–7 days to complete, resulting in the production of approximately 40,000 parasites per infecting sporozoite.

3  The mature tissue schizont ruptures its infected parenchymal cell and the merozoites enter the bloodstream. Merozoites only infect red cells. Hence reinvasion of the liver is not possible. Only a sporozoite transmitted by the bite of another infected mosquito can initiate a new exoerythrocytic cycle of division. No hypnozoites are formed by *P. falciparum*.

4a  Merozoites begin the erythrocytic cycle by invading red cells. With *P. facliparum* it is common to have more than one parasite in each red cell. This early stage of development is called the trophozoite and is commonly found in the peripheral circulation.

4b  Unlike the other three species of malaria that infect humans, *P. falciparum* develops beyond the trophozoite, inside red cells attached to endothelial cells lining the capillaries of the body, especially those in the deep tissues. The mechanisms by which this takes place apparently involve the parasite-directed elicitation of "knobs" on a portion of the infected red cell membrane. The physicochemical properties of these "knobs" together with other parasite-derived proteins enable them to bind to endothelial cell membrane. The attachment lasts throughout schizogony. The trophozoite grows within the immobilized infected red cell, feeding upon the protein portion of hemoglobin.

4c  Schizogony occurs every 48 hours and results in the production of 8 to 16 merozoites.

4d  The mature schizont breaks open, releasing its complement of merozoites.

4e  Noninfected red cells often become trapped in capillaries that harbor infected red cells.

4f  These trapped red cells are quickly infected by merozoites freed after schizogony. Gametocyte formation occurs in the peripheral circulation.

5a  The macrogametocyte is the female pre-sex cell.

5b  The microgametocyte is the male pre-sex cell.

5c  The female mosquito acquires her infection by ingesting both pre-sex cells along with a blood meal from an infected individual. There are no reservoir hosts for any species of human malaria.

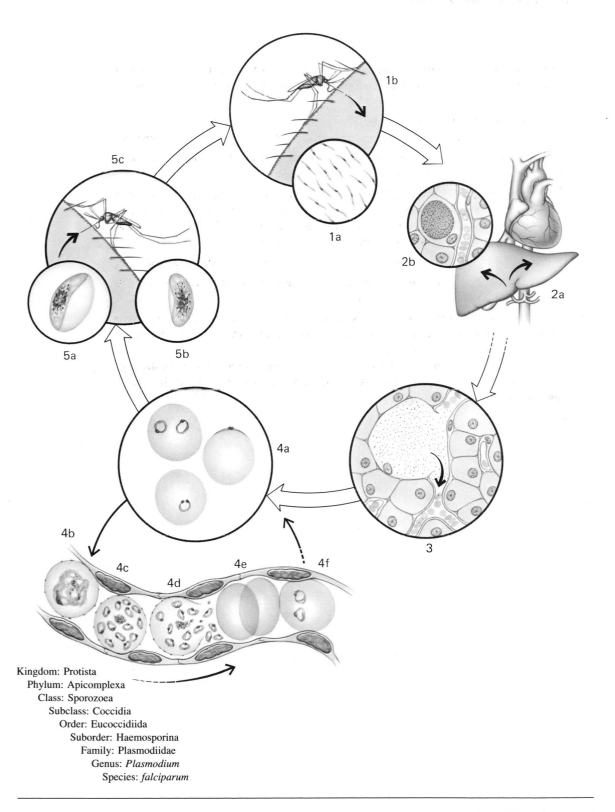

Kingdom: Protista
Phylum: Apicomplexa
Class: Sporozoea
Subclass: Coccidia
Order: Eucoccidiida
Suborder: Haemosporina
Family: Plasmodiidae
Genus: *Plasmodium*
Species: *falciparum*

# Balantidium Coli

1a    The infective stage for the human is the cyst. The cyst is 55 μm in diameter and is surrounded by a resistant thickened wall. Its cytoplasm contains a single micro- and macronucleus.

1b    The cyst must be ingested in order for the life cycle to begin. Food and water contaminated with feces from infected individuals serve as the sources of infection.

2    Excystment occurs in the small intestine, while the trophozoites reside in the large intestine. Each cyst produces a single trophozoite.

3a    The trophozoite is 70 μm long by 45 μm in width and is completely surrounded by cilia. Its cytoplasm contains a contractile vacuole, a single micronucleus, and a single cresent-shaped macronucleus. In addition, the trophozoite has a cytostome through which it ingests its food; namely, living host cells.

3b    It divides by binary fission within the walls of the submucosa of the large intestine.

4a    Encystation occurs in the lumen. The process results in the production of a thick wall that surrounds and protects the organism.

4b    Encystation is complete when the cyst wall is fully contiguous. Cysts pass into the environment with the fecal mass where they can remain infective for another host for extended periods of time.

5    Although other mammalian species, such as the Guinea pig and the domestic pig, can become infected with *B. coli,* it is not known if any of them are important reservoir hosts.

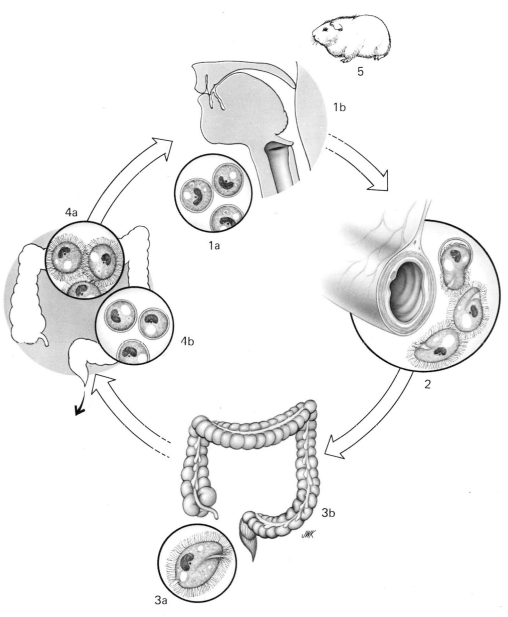

Kingdom: Protista
Phylum: Ciliophora
Class: Kinetofragminophorea
Subclass: Vestibuliferia
Order: Trichostomatida
Suborder: Trichostomatina
Family: Balantidiidae
Genus: *Balantidium*
Species: *coli*

# 2 Cestoidea

# General Characteristics of Cestodes

All adult cestodes (tapeworms) are parasitic and live within the digestive tract of their hosts. All vertebrates can harbor tapeworm adults, but only a few species of tapeworms infect the human host. Tapeworms vary greatly in size, with some achieving lengths of over 10 meters, while others grow only centimeters in length. Nearly all cestodes rely on intermediate hosts for transmission, which may in some cases be a mammal (e.g., *Taenia saginata* in the cow and *Taenia solium* in the pig).

The adult worm typically consists of a head (scolex) and a segmented body (strobila), each segment of which is termed a proglottid. None possesses a digestive tract; hence they absorb all nutrients through their outer surface (tegument).

The scolex attaches to the host epithelium by means of suckers, hooks, grooves, or a combination of these holdfast organs, depending upon the species in question. Proglottids are produced near the neck of the strobila and exhibit increasing degrees of maturation the further away from the scolex they are found. Finally, the last segments are those that contain fertilized eggs and usually detach from the colony of proglottids, or disintegrate, releasing their eggs into the lumen of the intestine. Eggs can either be eaten by an intermediate host and undergo further development, or hatch, infect an intermediate host, and then undergo morphogenesis to the next stage. Ultimately, the definitive host must ingest the infective larval tapeworm to acquire the infection.

The entire surface of the tegument is covered with small fingerlike projections (microtriches), which are thought to both aid in adherence of the worm to the intestinal surface, and to increase its own absorption surface. As already mentioned, all nutrients must be absorbed, either passively or actively through the tegument.

Below the tegument lies a complex arrangement of muscle, nerve, excretory, and reproductive tissues. The musculature runs both longitudinally and circularly. Their muscle cells lack T-tubules and are nonstriated. The excretory tubules run on either lateral side of each segment and transport wastes to the host intestinal lumen. Specialized ciliated cells called flame cells aid in fluid movement. The tegument and excretory system have been implicated in osmoregulation. The scolex possesses ganglia from which emanate various branches of nerves running the length of the strobila. The head may contain sensory nerves ending in specialized regions that aid the worm in seeking nutrient gradients. The nerves communicate via lateral commissures.

Each segment usually contains a complete set of male and female reproductive organs. As already mentioned the farther away from the scolex the segment is, the more sexually mature it is. Each proglottid makes a full complement of sperm and eggs. Often, the sperm are stored and self-fertilization in each proglottid occurs. However, segments can also exchange sperm. If two worms of the same species are present in the same host, they can mate with each other. Sperm are produced in the testes, which are connected to the vas efferens. Sperm are stored in the external seminal receptacle. The female system reproductive system consists of the ovary, vitelline glands, oviduct, and Mehlis' gland. Egg yolk is formed by the vitelline cells which join with the ovum to produce the unfertilized egg. Fertilization occurs when the egg passes through the oviduct. Meiosis is complete after fertilization. The vitelline membrane is then laid down and the zygote and/or vitelline cells secrete the eggshell, itself depending on the species. Embryonation then ensues, resulting in gravid proglottids, which may contain hundreds to thousands of infectious eggs.

# Classification

**Bold type** indicates orders represented in book by parasites

Kingdom: Animal
  Phylum: Platyhelminthes
    Class: Turbellaria
    Class: Monogenea
    Class: Trematoda
    Class: Cestoidea
      Subclass: Cestodaria
        Family: Amphilinidae
        Family: Austramphilinidae
        Family: Gyrocotylidae
      Subclass: Eucestoda
      Order: Caryophyllidea
        Family: Caryophyllaeidae
      Order: Spathebothriidea
        Family: Cyathocephalidae
        Family: Spathebothriidae
      Order: Trypanorhyncha
        Family: Dasyrhynchidae
        Family: Eutetrarhynchidae
        Family: Gilquiniidae
        Family: Gymnorhynchidae
        Family: Hepatoxylidae
        Family: Hornelliellidae
        Family: Lacistorhynchidae
        Family: Mustelicolidae
        Family: Otobothriidae
        Family: Paranybeliniidae
        Family: Pterobothriidae
        Family: Sphyriocephalidae
        Family: Tentaculariidae
      Order: Pseudophyllidea
        Family: Amphicotylidae
        Family: Bothriocephalidae
        Family: Cephalochlamydidae
        **Family: Diphyllobothriidae**
        Family: Echinophallidae
        Family: Haplobothriidae
        Family: Parabothriocephalidae

        Family: Ptychobothriidae
        Family: Triaenophoridae
      Order: Lecanicephalidea
        Family: Adelobothriidae
        Family: Balanobothriidae
        Family: Disculicepitidae
        Family: Lecanicephalidae
      Order: Aporidea
        Family: Nematoparataeniidae
      Order: Tetraphyllidea
        Family: Dioecotaeniidae
        Family: Onchobothriidae
        Family: Phyllobothriidae
        Family: Triloculariidae
      Order: Diphyllidea
        Family: Ditrachybathridiidae
        Family: Echinobothriidae
      Order: Litobothridea
        Family: Litobothridae
      Order: Proteocephalata
        Family: Proteocephalidae
      Order: Cyclophyllidea
        Family: Amabiliidae
        Family: Anoplocephalidae
        Family: Catenotaeniidae
        Family: Davaineidae
        **Family: Dilepididae**
        Family: Dioecocestidae
        Family: Diploposthidae
        **Family: Hymenolepididae**
        Family: Mesocestoididae
        Family: Nematotaeniidae
        Family: Progynotaeniidae
        **Family: Taeniidae**
        Family: Tetrabothriidae
        Family: Triplotaeniidae
      Order: Nippotaeniidea
        Family: Nippotaeniidae

# Diphyllobothrium Latum

1a  The infective stage for the human host of *D. latum* is the pleroceroid, which lives between the myomeres in muscle tissue of freshwater fish.

1b  The mode of infection is by oral ingestion of undercooked or raw unfrozen infected freshwater fish.

2a  Following ingestion, the pleurocercoid develops to the immature adult. The scolex of the adult worm attaches to the wall of the small intestine by means of two bilateral grooves called bothria.

2b  Differentiation, growth, and maturation occurs within the lumen of the small intestine.

3a  Hundreds of immature, mature, and gravid segments are produced within 20 days after ingestion of the pleurocercoid. Adult worms can achieve lengths exceeding 14 meters.

3b  The mature proglottid can be distinguished from other adult tapeworms infecting the human host by the fact that its birth pore exits from the center of the dorsal surface, rather than laterally.

4a  Gravid proglottids periodically release eggs into the lumen.

4b  The eggs become included within the fecal mass prior to being passed outside the host during defecation. It has been estimated that a large adult worm can produce some $10^6$ eggs each day.

4c  The unembryonated eggs have a single operculum and must be deposited in fresh water for continuation of the life cycle.

5a  After an incubation period of approximately 18–20 days, the operculated end of the egg opens, and the free-swimming coracidium emerges into the aquatic environment. This stage moves about aided by extremely long cilia covering its entire outer surface. The coracidium can survive for 12–14 hours as a free-swimming larva before it exhausts its stored energy supply and dies.

5b  The coracidium is able to develop to the next stage only after being ingested by crustaceans in the genus *Diaptomus*. After the coracidium is eaten, it penetrates the hemocoel of *Diaptomus* and transforms into the procercoid stage over a 2- to 3-week period.

5c  Minnows and other small fish feed upon both infected and noninfected Diaptomus. If an infected *Diaptomus* is eaten, then the procercoid is released from the crustacean, penetrates the fish's small intestine, and finally migrates to between the myomeres. There it develops to the plerocercoid, the infective stage for the human host.

5d  Humans do not usually eat raw or undercooked minnows, and therefore these infected smaller fish do not serve as important vectors for the infection. However, if an infected minnow is eaten by a larger predator species of fish (e.g., trout, walleyed pike, Northern pike, or perch), then the pleurocercoid can relocate between the myomeres of the musculature of the larger fish. Hence transmission of the infection is through the ingestion of these latter intermediate hosts.

6  Bears can serve as reservoir hosts for *Diphyllobothrium latum*.

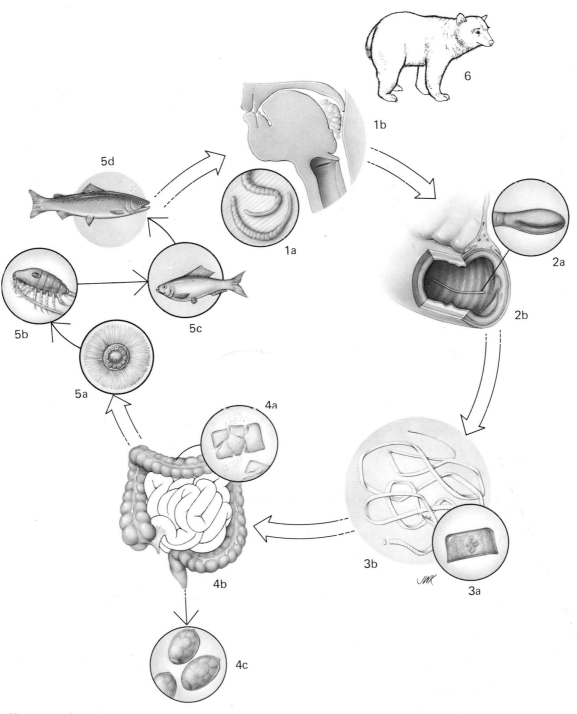

6

5d

1b

1a

2a

2b

5b

5c

5a

4a

3b

3a

4b

4c

Kingdom: Animal
Phylum: Platyhelminthes
Class: Cestoidea
Order: Pseudophyllidea
Family: Diphyllobothriidae
Genus: *Diphyllobothrium*
Species: *latum*

# Dipylidium Caninum

1   The infective stage of *Dipylidium caninum* is the cysticercoid (6b) and lives within the haemocoel of the dog flea, *Ctenocephalides canis*. The infected flea must be ingested to initiate infection in the human host.

2   The flea's tissues are digested away from the cysticercoid in the stomach and small intestine.

3a   The hook-studded scolex of *D. caninum* attaches to the wall of the small intestine.

3b   In approximately 20–25 days, the worm matures to adulthood within the lumen of the small intestine.

4a   The adult of *D. caninum* is 30–40 cm in length, but can achieve a length of over 70 cm.

4b   The characteristic proglottid has two genital pores, each of which opens laterally on either side of the segment.

5a   Gravid proglottids break off from the parent colony and pass out, *intact,* in the feces.

5b   The packets of eggs contained within each proglottid are held together by an outer embryonic membrane. The proglottids disintegrate in the soil, releasing the packets of eggs.

6a   The eggs must then be ingested by the larvae of fleas to continue the life cycle. The eggs hatch within the flea's midgut, and the hexacanth tapeworm larva migrates into the hemocoel, where it transforms into the cysticercoid.

6b   The cysticercoid is retained by the flea during its own morphogenesis to an adult insect.

6c   The adult flea, harboring the cysticercoid, must now be ingested by the definitive mammalian host for the life cycle to become complete.

7   Dog is the usual definitive host for this tapeworm. The cysticercoid is usually ingested together with the infected flea (i.e., the intermediate host).

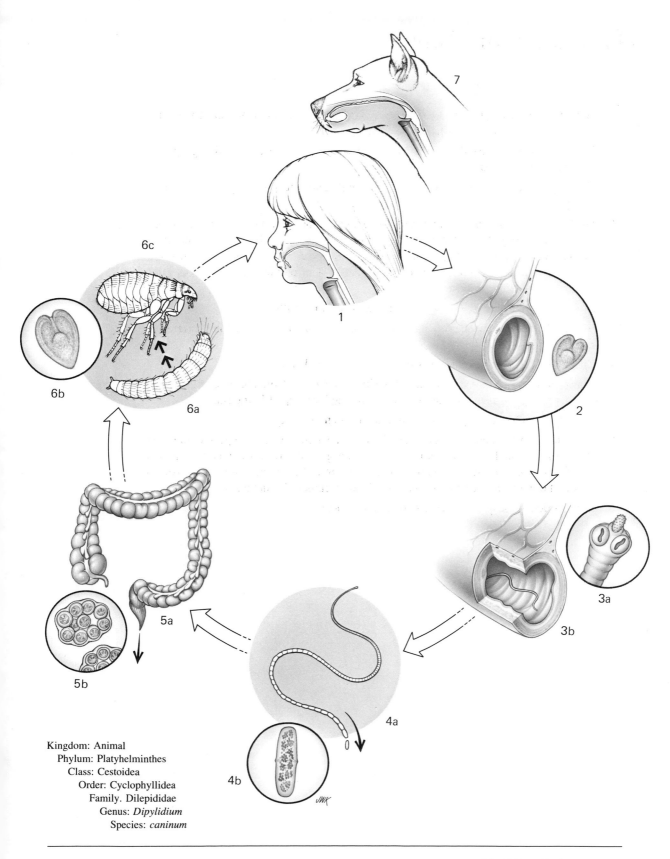

Kingdom: Animal
 Phylum: Platyhelminthes
  Class: Cestoidea
   Order: Cyclophyllidea
    Family. Dilepididae
     Genus: *Dipylidium*
      Species: *caninum*

# Hymenolepis Nana

1a  The embryonated egg of *Hymenolepis nana* contains polar filaments, thereby distinguishing it from that of *Hymenolepis diminuta*.

1b  The egg can be ingested directly by the definitive host. Feces containing eggs is the source of infection.

2  The eggs hatch within the lumen of the small intestine releasing the hexacanth embryo.

3  The hexacanth embryo penetrates the villus tissue of the small intestine and develops into the cysticeroid. Alternatively, eggs can be ingested by the intermediate host, various beetles species, and proceed to develop to cysticercoids within the hemocoel, as with *H. diminuta*. Thus, *H. nana* can infect its definitive host directly or through an intermediate insect host.

4a  In the direct life cycle, the cysticercoid exits from the villus.

4b  Within 6 days it attaches to the wall of the lumen of the small intestine after everting the scolex.

5a  The scolex of *H. nana* possesses both hooks and suckers.

5b  Maturation to the adult stage takes approximately 30 days from the time of ingestion of the egg and 5 days less than that if an infected arthropod is ingested.

6a  The proglottid of *H. nana* has a single lateral genital pore.

6b  The adult worm measures about 30–40 cm in length. Eggs are passed into the lumen of the small intestine either through the genital atrium of gravid segments or are released after such proglottids break off from the parent colony and disintegrate. The eggs are passed into the outside environment by defecation.

7  Small rodents are the most common reservoir hosts.

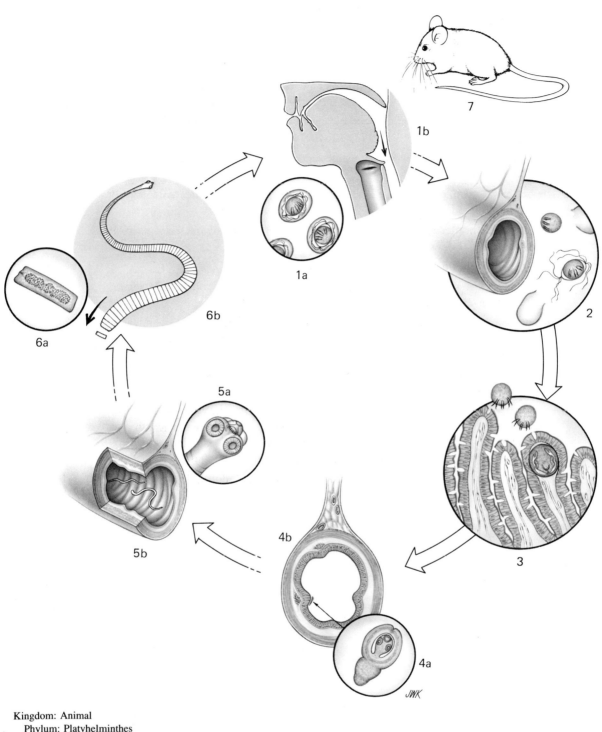

Kingdom: Animal
  Phylum: Platyhelminthes
    Class: Cestoidea
      Order: Cyclophyllidea
        Family: Hymenolepididae
          Genus: *Hymenolepis*
            Species: *nana*

# Hymenolepis Diminuta

1a  The intermediate host is usually a coleopteran in the genus *Tribolium*. However, various other genera of beetles can also serve this function in the life cycle.

1b  The beetle, infected with the cysticerocid larva of *H. diminuta,* must be ingested in order to initiate infection with this cestode.

2  The tissues of the infected beetle are digested away from the cysticercoids in the stomach and small intestine.

3a  The scolex, which possesses four suckers, everts from the cysticercoid shortly after being released from the beetle.

3b  The scolex then attaches to the wall of the lumen of the small intestine where it matures within 20 days.

4a  The gravid proglottid has a single lateral genital pore.

4b  The adult worm is small in length compared to the *Taenia* spp. or *D. latum,* achieving an average length of 30 cm.

5a  The eggs are passed out the genital atrium of gravid segments, or are released into the lumen of the small intestine when egg-laden segments break off from the parent colony and disintegrate.

5b  Eggs thus released are included into the fecal mass and are passed out of the host during defecation.

6a  The eggs become ingested by the larvae of *Tribolium* spp. beetles and other Coleoptera. In the insect's small intestine, the egg hatches, releasing the hexacanth embryo. The embryo then penetrates the intestinal tract and eventually transforms into the cysticercoid (i.e., the infective stage for the definitive host) in the hemocoel.

6b  The cysticercoid survives the insect's morphogenesis to an adult arthropod.

7  While humans often become infected with *H. diminuta,* it is more commonly a parasite of rodents, such as rats and mice.

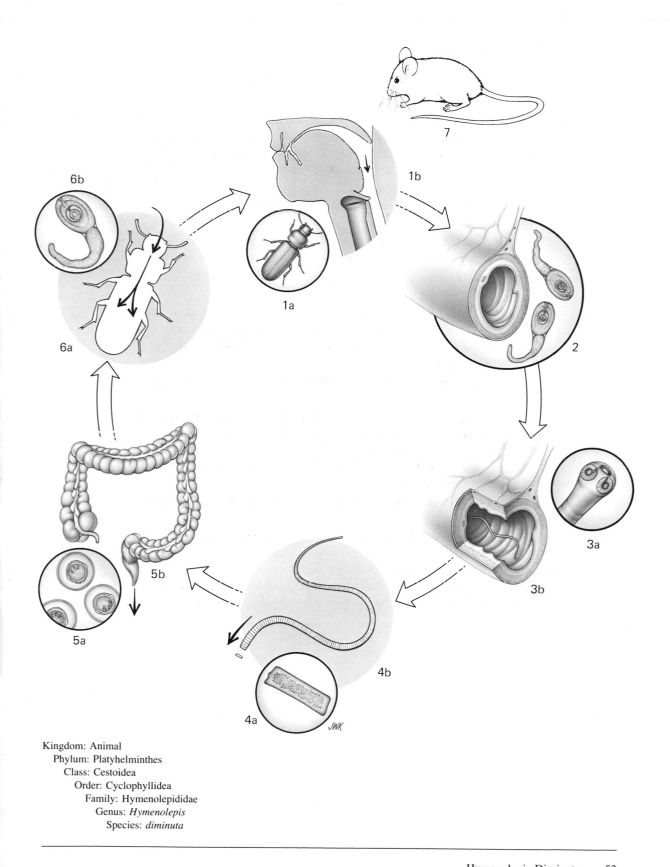

Kingdom: Animal
Phylum: Platyhelminthes
Class: Cestoidea
Order: Cyclophyllidea
Family: Hymenolepididae
Genus: *Hymenolepis*
Species: *diminuta*

# Taenia Saginata

1a  The infective stage for the human (i.e., definitive) host is the juvenile worm termed the cysticercus. No other mammal can serve as the definitive host for this tapeworm. The cysticercus lives encysted within the tissues of the intermediate host, the cow. All bovine tissues may harbor cysticerci, but skeletal muscle is the most common source of infection.

1b  The cysticercus must be ingested in raw or undercooked unfrozen beef for the life cycle to begin within the human host.

2  The cysticerci are digested away from the tissues of the cow in the stomach. The freed cysticerci enter the small intestine and initiate development toward adulthood.

3a  In the small intestine, the immature tapeworm evaginates its scolex (note the absence of hooks).

3b  The scolex attaches to the inner wall of the small intestine by means of its four suckers, and in approximately 8–12 weeks develops into a fully mature worm. An adult *T. saginata* can grow to as long as 10 meters, but 6 meters is typical.

4a  The gravid proglottid contains some 100,000 eggs. The uterus has more than 12 branches on each side, thereby distinguishing it from that of *T. solium* (see Figure 4a, page 57).

4b  Gravid proglottids break off from the parent colony and pass live through the anus to the external environment. During its passage through the anal sphincter, some eggs may be expressed from the proglottid and come to rest on the perianal region of the host. Eggs may be expelled from the *intact* parent colony, but this is an uncommon mode of egg dispersal.

5a  The embryonated eggs become liberated from the proglottids when the segments disintegrate in the soil.

5b  Ingestion of embryonated eggs by cattle results in their hatching within the small intestine. The hexacanth larvae then penetrate the bloodstream and are carried to various organs throughout the body, including brain, eye, skeletal musculature, and the heart. There, within 2 months, the larvae develop into cysticerci, the infective stage for the human host. There are no reservoir hosts for *Taenia saginata*.

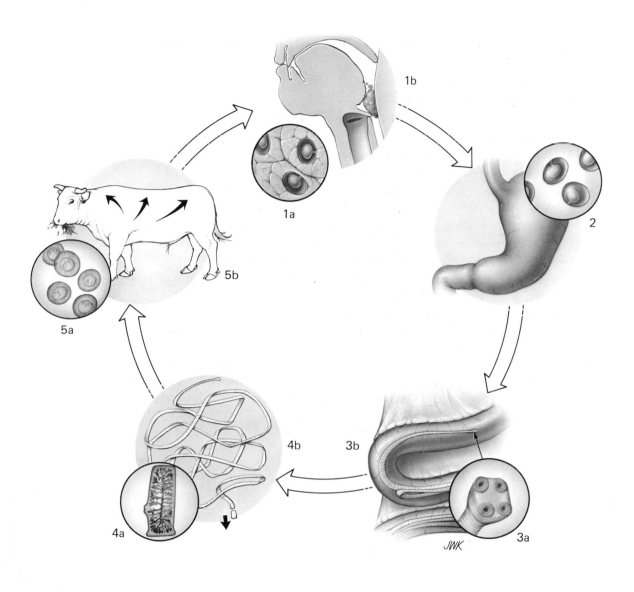

Kingdom: Animal
  Phylum: Platyhelminthes
    Class: Cestoidea
      Order: Cyclophyllidea
        Family: Taeniidae
          Genus: *Taenia*
            Species: *saginata*

# Taenia Solium

1a  The stage leading to adult tapeworm infection for the human host is the cysticercus (i.e., juvenile tapeworm).

1b  The cysticercus, together with a portion of infected undercooked or raw unfrozen pork must be ingested in order to begin the cycle.

2  Cysticerci are liberated from muscle tissue in the stomach. The freed cysticerci then enter the small intestine by peristalsis.

3a  The scolex evaginates and attaches to the wall of the small intestine. It utilizes both hooks and suckers to remain there.

3b  The worm matures within the lumen of the small intestine over a period of 10–12 weeks.

4a  The adult worm averages 4 meters in length. The gravid proglottids break off from the parent colony and actively migrate out the anus to the external environment. More rarely, groups of proglottids break off and are passed out with the feces.

4b  The gravid proglottid, containing thousands of eggs, has less than 10 uterine branches per side, thereby distinguishing it from that of *T. saginata* (see page 54).

5a  The embryonated eggs are infectious for the pig (i.e., the intermediate host) upon being passed from the human host in feces. Humans can also become infected with the larval form.

5b  After the pig ingests the eggs, they hatch in the small intestine; the hexacanth larvae penetrate the gut and enter the bloodstream and are carried to various organs throughout the body where they encyst and develop to cysticerci. Development to this stage after penetrating a given organ takes about 3–5 weeks. The cysticerci are then infectious for the definitive host.

6  No other mammal can harbor the adult of *T. solium*.

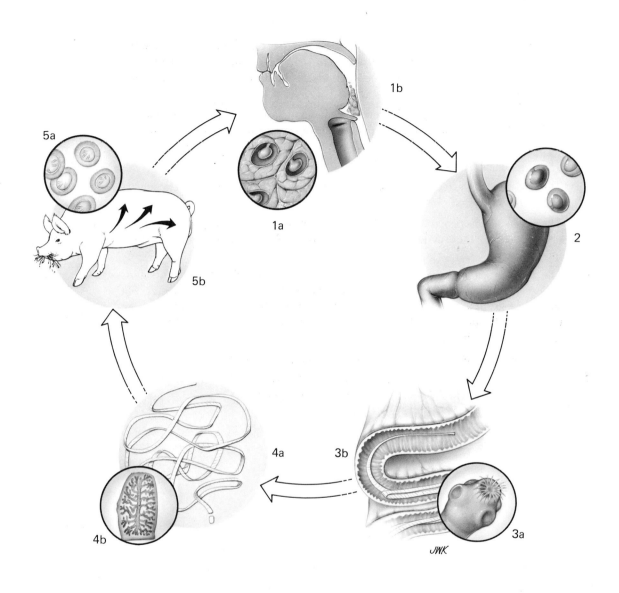

Kingdom: Animal
Phylum: Platyhelminthes
Class: Cestoidea
Order: Cyclophyllidea
Family: Taeniidae
Genus: *Taenia*
Species: *solium*

# Taenia Solium (Cysticercosis)

1a  The infectious stage for the intermediate host is the egg. The pig is the usual intermediate host (see life cycle for the adult stage of *Taenia solium*). However, humans can also harbor the juvenile stage of *T. solium* if they ingest eggs rather than cysticerci (i.e., the juvenile stage).

1b  Ingestion of eggs initiates the infection. Food and inanimate objects contaminated with feces from humans harboring the adult tapeworm are the usual sources of infection.

2a  The eggs hatch in the small intestine.

2b  The oncosphere (hexacanth larva) is stimulated to hatch when the egg encounters bile salts in the small intestine.

3  The oncospheres penetrate into the bloodstream and are carried to a variety of organs. There, they undergo extensive growth and development, transforming into cysticerci.

4a-d  The cysticercus is ovoid in shape and measures approximately 10 mm at its widest point (4a). A variety of organs can become infected with cysticerci, but subcutaneous tissue is the most common site invaded. The cysticerci lodge between the muscle bundles (4b). The eye (4c) and brain (4d) are other common sites of larval *T. solium* infection.

5a  The adult worm in the human host is the source of infectious eggs.

5b  The eggs are found within gravid proglottids of the adult worm and pass into the environment when defecated proglottids disintegrate.

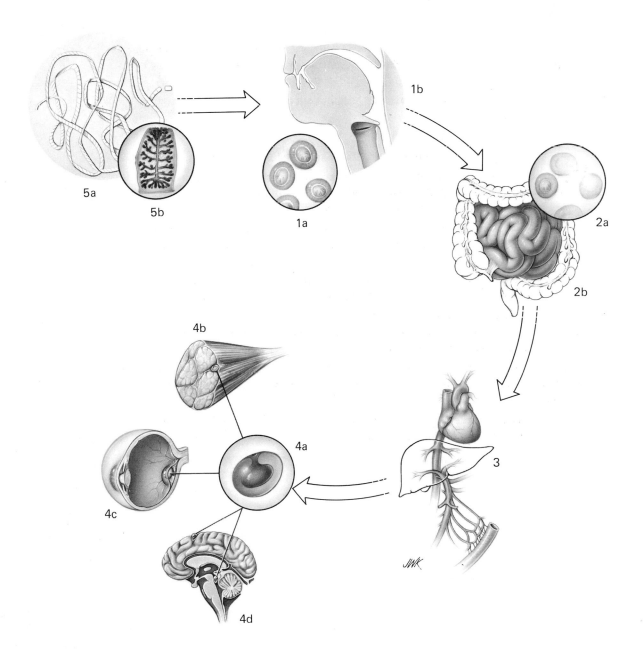

# Taenia Multiceps

1a  The embryonated eggs are infectious for a wide variety of mammals, including sheep (5c) and humans. Feces containing eggs from infected dogs is the source of infection.

1b  The eggs are ingested by the intermediate host through contamination of the environment by dog feces.

2  Hatching occurs in the small intestine.

3a  The hexacanth larva is morphologically similar to all taeniid tapeworm species.

3b  The hexacanth larva (35 μm in diameter) penetrates the small intestine and enters the bloodstream via the portal system and is carried to any one of a variety of organs within the body. There it develops to the next stage, the coenurus.

4a  The brain (shown in coronal section) is a common site for the coenurus to develop. The coenurus is a large fluid-filled cyst that grows to an average diameter of 35 mm.

4b  Inside the coenurus, the germinal layer gives rise to infectious units termed protoscolices, each of which is capable of developing to an adult in the definitive host.

5a  The dog and other carnivores serve as definitive hosts of *T. multiceps*. They acquire their infection through the ingestion of coenuri. This usually occurs when dogs are fed infected organs of slaughtered sheep.

5b  Adult worms develop within the dog's small intestine. After the worms mature, embryonated eggs are passed in the feces and become ingested by sheep and, occasionally, humans.

5c  The sheep is a common intermediate host for *T. multiceps*. In the human the parasite's life cycle is considered aberrant.

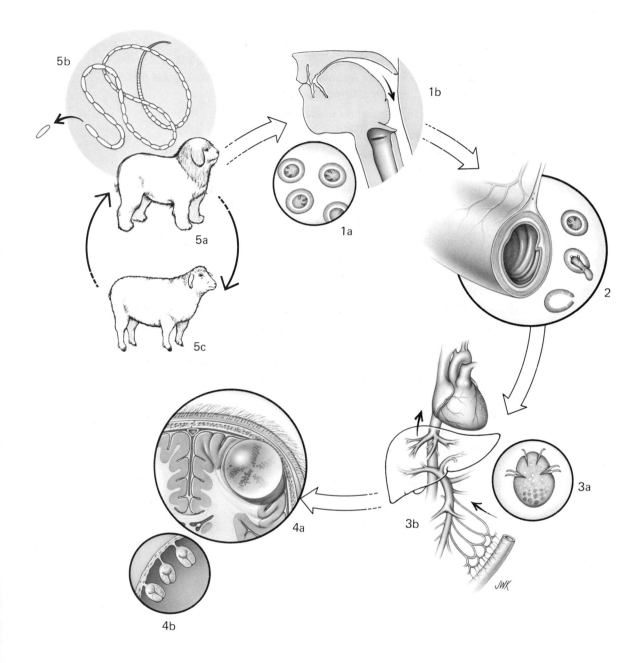

Kingdom: Animal
  Phylum: Platyhelminthes
    Class: Cestoidea
      Order: Cyclophyllidea
       Family: Taeniidae
         Genus: *Taenia*
           Species: *multiceps*

# Echinococcus Granulosus

1a  The embryonated eggs are infectious for the intermediate hosts, which include various ruminants and humans. Food and inanimate objects contaminated with dog feces containing eggs are the most common source of infection. In many parts of the world, sheep are the most common intermediate host.

1b  The eggs must be ingested to begin infection in the human host.

2  Hatching occurs in the small intestine.

3a  The hexacanth larva, referred to as the oncosphere, is typical of all tapeworm larvae, possessing six hookletes.

3b  Through the use of its hookletes, the oncosphere penetrates the wall of the intestinal tract and enters the portal system. Usually, the oncosphere penetrates the liver where it transforms into the cyst stage. More rarely, other organs are infected.

4a  The cyst takes several months to mature, becoming thin-walled and filled with fluid, hence the term "hydatid cyst." Its average diameter at maturity can be as much as 30 cm. In the brain the size of the cyst is much less, since the space limitations of the cranium do not permit further expansion.

4b  The wall of the hydatid cyst consists of an outer acellular laminate membrane and an inner cellular germinal layer. The protoscolices are produced by budding from the inner surface of the germinal layer.

4c  Small packets of protoscolices, referred to as brood capsules, may contain as many as 6 to 12 protoscolices. Each protoscolex, if ingested, can develop into an adult worm in the definitive host.

5a  Canines, particularly domestic dogs, serve as definitive hosts for *E. granulosus*. They usually acquire their infection by ingesting organs of slaughtered sheep or reindeer which harbor the hydatid cyst.

5b  Thousands of adult worms may develop in the intestinal tract of the dog after the ingestion of a single large, mature hydatid cyst.

5c  Sheep acquire their cysts from ingestion of eggs passed in the feces of infected dogs. The eggs are passed in an embryonated state and are immediately infectious.

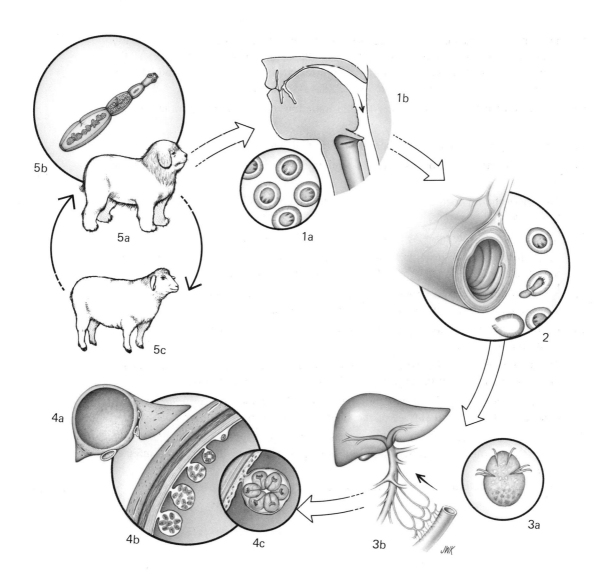

Kingdom: Animal
  Phylum: Platyhelminthes
    Class: Cestoidea
      Order: Cyclophyllidea
        Family: Taeniidae
          Genus: *Echinococcus*
            Species: *granulosus*

# Echinococcus Multilocularis

1a  The embryonated egg is the infectious stage for the intermediate host, usually small rodents. Feces containing eggs from the definitive host (e.g., fox) is the source of infection. Humans who become infected resemble intermediate hosts in regard to the stage of the life cycle which develops after infection.

1b  Ingestion of the eggs is necessary for the initiation of infection in the intermediate host.

2  The oncosphere hatches from the egg in the small intestine.

3a  The hexacanth larva (oncosphere) is similar in morphology to all other cestode oncospheres.

3b  The oncosphere penetrates the small intestine, enters the bloodstream and is carried to the liver.

4a  In the vole and human hosts, the multilocular cyst develops in the liver.

4b  In the human, no protoscolices develop. Rather, only the laminate acellular outer membrane and the inner germinal layer can be demonstrated.

4c  Viable protoscolices are produced within each compartment of the cyst. Protoscolex development only occurs in the vole and related rodent species.

4d  Each protoscolex is produced from the inner surface of the germinal layer within each compartment.

5a  The definitive host is the fox (and related carnivores in the family Caniidae), acquiring its worms through the ingestion of the infected intermediate host.

5b  The adult worm, similar in morphology to that of *Echinococcus granulosus,* lives attached to the luminal surface of the small intestine of the definitive host.

5c  The vole serves as the most important intermediate host for *E. multilocularis,* and acquires its infection through ingesting the eggs passed in the feces of infected foxes.

6  Dogs are the definitive hosts for *Echinococcus granulosus.*

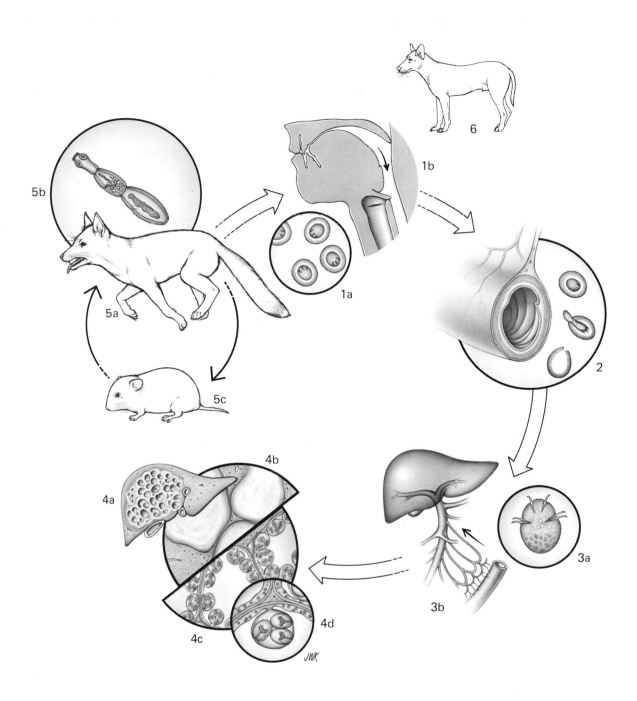

Kingdom: Animal
　Phylum: Platyhelminthes
　　Class: Cestoidea
　　　Order: Cyclophyllidea
　　　　Family: Taeniidae
　　　　　Genus: *Echinococcus*
　　　　　　Species: *multilocularis*

# 3 Trematoda

# General Characteristics of Trematodes

All adult trematodes in the subclass Digenea, commonly referred to as flukes, are parasitic, occupying a wide variety of sites within the human host. Some live within the lumen of organs, while others infect solid tissue, such as liver and lung.

The nonsegmented adult worms vary greatly in morphology, depending upon the species. There are two distinct types: one in which the sexes are separate (e.g., Family Schistosomatidae), and the other in which both sets of reproductive organs are found within the same individual. In the latter group (i.e., the majority of Families within the Subclass Digenea), self- or cross-fertilization may occur, while the schistosomes require both sexes for egg production. Both groups of flukes are surrounded by a tegument whose surface contains various projections and spines. Nutrients are obtained by active transport of small molecular weight substances across the tegument and by ingestion and digestion of host tissues. The products of digestion are absorbed across the gut wall and enter the parenchymal tissues of the worm. The source of nutrients varies greatly for each worm species, and is largely determined by the worms' location within each host. Each adult worm has two suckers, one anterior and one ventral. The suckers are multipurposed, serving functions related to attachment and movement.

Below the level of the tegument lie the parenchymal, muscle, nerve, excretory, and reproductive systems.

Eggs may be produced either embryonated or nonembryonated, depending upon the species in question. In all cases, eggs must eventually exit from the host. The male reproductive organs typically consist of the testes, vas deferens and the external seminal vesicle and cirrus. The female reproductive system includes the ovary, vitelline cells, Mehlis' gland, oviduct, uterus and metraterm. Eggs, in an advanced state of embryogenesis, leave the ovary, pass down the oviduct, acquire yolk, and are fertilized. The eggshell is produced by the vitelline cells. Eventually, the eggs exit from the genital pore and must pass out of the host into an aquatic environment for the life cycle to continue. All trematodes utilize snails as their first intermediate host. Within the snail, the worm undergoes remarkable changes, both in morphology and in numbers, resulting in infectious larvae, which exit from the snail and either encyst or penetrate the human host to complete their life cycle. Those species that encyst usually do so on plants or on invertebrates or vertebrates. Often, the second intermediate host is an amphibian. Thus, these flukes must be eaten in order to carry out their life cycles.

# Classification

**Bold type** indicates superfamilies represented in book by parasites

Kingdom: Animal
  Phylum: Platyhelminthes
    Class: Cestoidea
    Class: Turbellaria
    Class: Monogenea
    Class: Trematoda
      Subclass: Digenea
        Superorder: Anepitheliocystidia
          Order: Strigeata
            Superfamily: Strigeoidea
            Superfamily: Clinostomatoidea
            **Superfamily: Schistosomatoidea**
            Superfamily: Azygioidea
            Superfamily: Transversotrematoidea
            Superfamily: Cyclocoeloidea
            Superfamily: Brachylaemoidea
            Superfamily: Fellodistomatoidea
            Superfamily: Bucephaloidea
          Order: Echinostomata
            **Superfamily: Echinostomatoidea**
            Superfamily: Paramphistomoidea
            Superfamily: Notocotyloidea
        Superorder: Epitheliocystidia
          Order: Plagiorchiata
            Superfamily: Plagiorchioidea
            **Superfamily: Allocreadioidea**
          Order: Opisthorchiata
            Superfamily: Isoparorchioidea
            **Superfamily: Opisthorchioidea**
            Superfamily: Hemiuroidea

# Schistosoma Mansoni

1   The cercaria penetrates the skin at the level of the hair follicle thereby initiating infection. The forked tail is lost during penetration, and the worm is now referred to as a schistosomula. The schistosomula penetrates the dermis, where it undergoes further development over the next several days. The schistosomule then migrates to the lungs, undergoing morphogenic changes there, as well.

2a   It is not known how schistosomules reach the liver, but the hematogenous route is the most likely one.

2b   Following maturity within the capillaries of the liver, mating ensues. The surface of the adult male is covered with small knoblike protuberances. Adults are 12 mm in length and 2 mm in diameter. Each worm has an anterior and ventral sucker with which it attaches to endothelial cells.

3   Pairs of worms migrate within the portal circulation, finally residing in the mesenteric venules of the small intestine. The female begins to lay eggs shortly after arriving there. Eggs exit from the genital pore, which is applied to the surface of the venule. Each female produces about 300 eggs per day.

4a   The egg contains the larval stage termed the miracidium. The miracidium secretes proteases which facilitates its penetration through venule endothelial cells, the connective tissue and the wall of the small intestine. Nearly 50% of the eggs reach the lumen of the small intestine. The other 50% are swept back into the presinusoidal capillaries of the liver where they no longer participate in the life cycle.

4b   Eggs are 110 μm long by 60 μm wide and possess a unique lateral spine.

5   Eggs reaching the lumen of the small intestine are passed from the host during defecation, and must be deposited in fresh water in which the appropriate snail host lives if the life cycle is to continue.

6a   The miracidium hatches from the egg in fresh water. This ciliated stage swims about seeking its snail host.

6b   The miracidium penetrates the snail. The most common vector snail species throughout tropical Central and South America is *Biomphalaria glabrata*. Other susceptible species of *Biomphalaria* occur in Africa. The trematode reaches the snail's hepatopancreas where it undergoes a series of morphogenic changes and then multiplies, transforming first into larvae termed sporocysts, then multiplying further into second-generation sporocysts. Secondary sporocysts give rise to many cercariae, the infectious stage for the human host.

6c   The phototropic cercariae exit from the snail and swim toward the surface of the water, aided by their forked tails. Cercariae live for about a day, then die if a host is not found.

7   Monkeys of various species can serve as reservoir hosts.

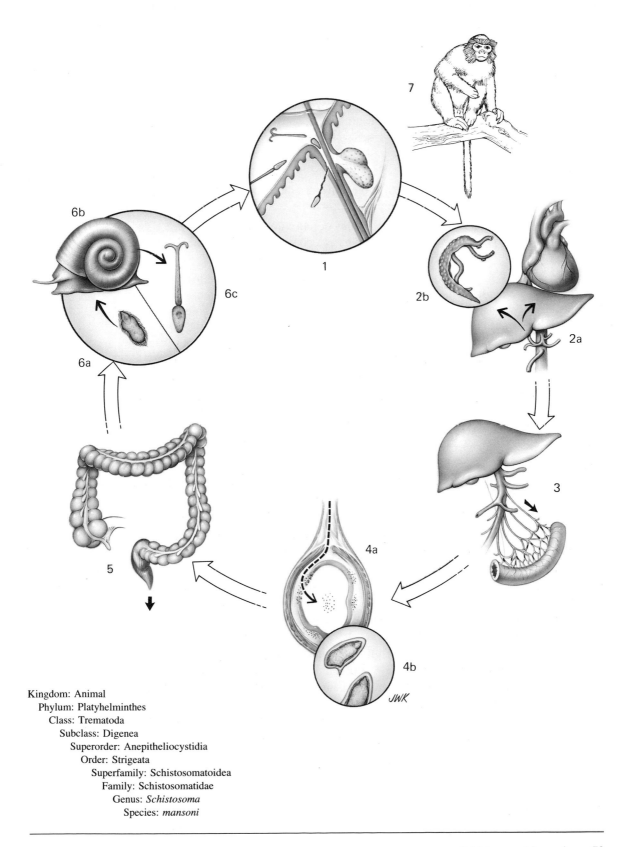

Kingdom: Animal
  Phylum: Platyhelminthes
    Class: Trematoda
      Subclass: Digenea
        Superorder: Anepitheliocystidia
          Order: Strigeata
            Superfamily: Schistosomatoidea
              Family: Schistosomatidae
                Genus: *Schistosoma*
                  Species: *mansoni*

# Schistosoma Japonicum

1   The fork-tailed cercaria penetrates the unbroken skin of the human host at the level of the hair follicle. Upon penetration, it loses its tail and burrows into the dermis. It is now referred to as a schistosomula. The schistosomula undergoes development there for several days, after which it migrates to the lungs, probably by the hematogenous route.

2a  The lung schistosomule develops further toward adulthood, then migrates to the liver, but the route taken by the lung schistosomule is not known.

2b  Maturation to an adult and subsequent mating occurs within the liver. The tegumental surface of *S. japonicum* adults is smooth, as opposed to either *S. mansoni* or *S. haematobium*. The adults are about 15 mm long and 0.5 mm wide.

3   Paired adults migrate out into the portal circulation against the flow of blood. Most of the adult worms locate in the mesenteric venules, but some may take up residence in the venules draining the spinal column or the brain. Those that locate in the mesenteric venules produce eggs that are able to continue the life cycle, while eggs produced in the other above-mentioned sites become sequestered in the capillaries. Each female worm produces about 2,000–3,000 eggs each day.

4a  Eggs laid up against the endothelium of the mesenteric venules penetrate into the surrounding connective tissue and eventually migrate into the lumen of the small intestine, aided by enzymes produced by the miracidia within them.

4b  Each *S. japonicum* egg is about 90 μm by 70 μm, is ovoid in shape, and has a small curved spine on its outer surface. Each egg has a ciliated miracidium within it.

5   Eggs that reach the lumen of the small intestine are included within the fecal mass and exit from the host during defecation. Eggs must reach fresh water in which an appropriate snail host lives in order for the life cycle to continue.

6a  Hatching occurs within 1 hour after the embryonated egg comes in contact with fresh water. The miracidium emerges and swims rapidly about seeking its intermediate snail host. Each miracidium is either male or female.

6b  The most common snail hosts for *S. japonicum* are in the genus *Oncomelania*. The miracidium penetrates the fleshy tissue of the snail and transforms at the site of penetration into the primary sporocyst. The primary sporocyst gives rise to many secondary sporocysts through repeated division cycles termed polyembryony.

6c  The secondary sporocysts in turn, give rise to the cercariae, the infectious stage for the mammalian host. The cercariae penetrate out of the snail and swim to the surface of the water, where they must encounter an appropriate mammalian host if the cycle is to be completed.

7   Primates of all species are susceptible to *S. japonicum* and many nonhuman primates serve as reservoir hosts for human infection.

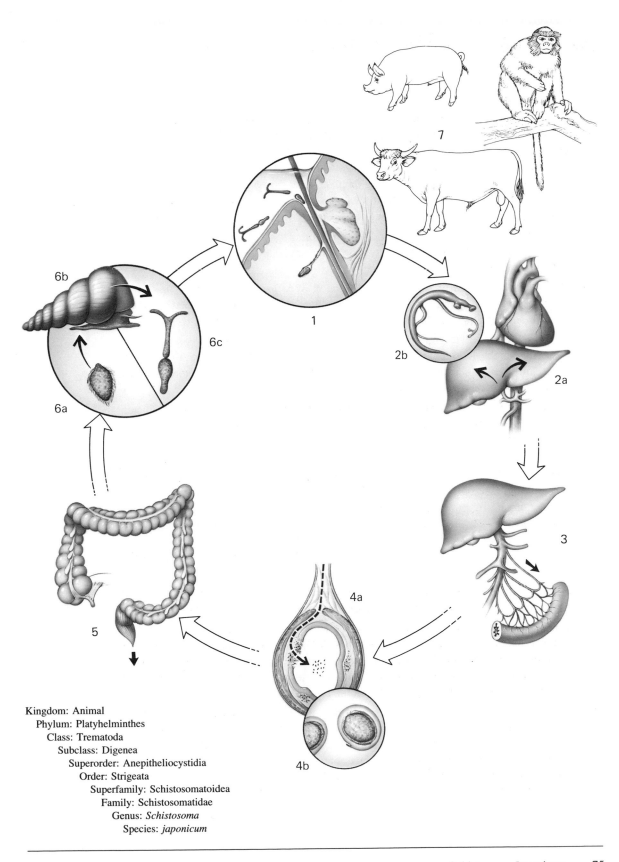

Kingdom: Animal
 Phylum: Platyhelminthes
  Class: Trematoda
   Subclass: Digenea
    Superorder: Anepitheliocystidia
     Order: Strigeata
      Superfamily: Schistosomatoidea
       Family: Schistosomatidae
        Genus: *Schistosoma*
         Species: *japonicum*

# Schistosoma Haematobium

1    The cercaria initiates the infection in the human host by penetrating the unbroken skin at the level of the hair follicle. Usually the area of skin most frequently penetrated is that which is at the surface of the water. The forked tail is lost upon entering the follicle; thus the cercaria transforms into the schistosomula. This stage penetrates into the dermis and, during the next several days, undergoes development toward adulthood. Subsequently, the skin schistosomule migrates to the lungs, probably via the hematogenous route, and undergoes further morphogenesis.

2a    From the lungs, the immature blood fluke migrates to the liver, where it completes its development into an adult trematode. The sexes are separate. Mating occurs within the blood vessels of the liver.

2b    The adults remain *in copula* for life. The adult of *S. haematobium* measures about 12 mm long and 1 mm wide. The protuberances on the male of *S. haematobium* are not as prominent as those found on the tegumental surface of *S. mansoni*.

3    The mature flukes migrate, as mated pairs, from the liver to the venous plexus surrounding the bladder, where the female worm begins her production of eggs. Eggs are produced in an embryonated state. It is not known how many eggs are produced each day by each female worm.

4a    The eggs of *Schistosoma haematobium* measure 140 μm by 60 μm and are characterized by an external terminal spine. The miracidium (i.e., the ciliated larva) lies within the egg.

4b    The adult female lays her eggs up against the endothelial cells of the venule. The miracidium within the egg secretes lytic enzymes which allows the egg to penetrate through the vessel wall and eventually through the smooth muscle wall of the bladder itself. Eggs reaching the lumen of the bladder are voided with the urine. About 50% of all eggs laid reach the lumen of the bladder. The rest wash back into the venous return and are trapped in the liver and, to a lesser extent, the lungs. These eggs do not exit from the host, and hence do not participate in the life cycle.

5a    Hatching occurs in fresh water. The ciliated miracidium swims about seeking its appropriate snail intermediate host. Various species of *Bulinus* serve in this capacity.

5b    The miracidium, upon finding a *Bulinus* snail, penetrates it and migrates to the hepatopancreas where the worm undergoes further development. Each miracidum is either male or female. This stage develops further, via division, into many sporocysts, then into secondary sporocysts. Each secondary sporocyst gives rise to many cercariae, the infectious stage for the human host.

5c    The forked tail cercariae penetrate out of the snail and immediately begin seeking out their human host. As with all other species of schistosomes, the cercaria of *S. haematobium* is positively phototactic and negatively geotropic, thus ensuring that it will quickly rise to the water's surface. If it does not find a host within 2 days, it loses its infectivity and dies shortly thereafter.

6    Non-human primates serve as reservoir hosts for *S. haematobium*.

---

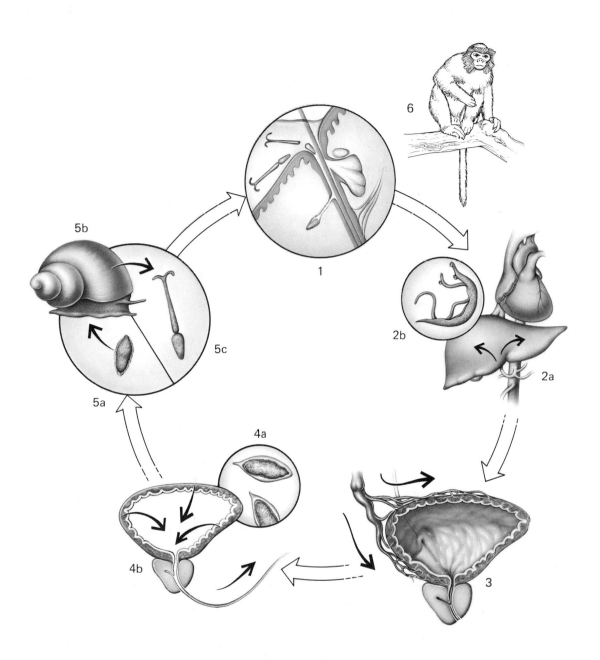

Kingdom: Animal
  Phylum: Platyhelminthes
    Class: Trematoda
      Subclass: Digenea
        Superorder: Anepitheliocystidia
          Order: Strigeata
            Superfamily: Schistosomatoidea
              Family: Schistosomatidae
                Genus: *Schistosoma*
                  Species: *haematobium*

# Fasciola Hepatica

1    Infection in the human host is initiated by swallowing the metacercaria (encysted larva) together with contaminated watercress or other littoral plants.

2    The metacercaria excysts within the lumen of the small intestine.

3    The immature fluke burrows through the wall of the small intestine, enters the peritoneal cavity, and penetrates the liver, where it then begins to feed upon the parenchymal cells. *Fasciola hepatica* grows slowly, achieving sexual maturity after 2 months in the liver. Fasciola is hermaphroditic, and self-mating may occur. Eggs are produced by each worm after another month of development.

4a    The adult flukes are among the largest that infect the human host. Each adult measure 25–30 mm in length and about 10–15 mm in width.

4b    Eggs are laid unembryonated within the tunnels created by the feeding worms in the liver tissue. The eggs reach the lumen of the small intestine by way of the hepatic ducts and, eventually, the common bile duct.

4c    Each egg measures approximately 115–120 $\mu$m in length by 55–60 $\mu$m in width and has an operculum at one end. The egg contains a single cell surrounded by yolk material. The egg exits from the host in the feces and must be deposited in fresh water to embryonate. Hatching takes place within 10–15 days after entering its aquatic environment.

5a    The ciliated miracidium swims about seeking its appropriate snail host. Upon encountering it, the miracidium penetrates the snail and develops within snail tissue.

5b    Snails in the genera *Lymnaea, Stagnicola,* and *Fossaria* serve as intermediate hosts for *Fasciola hepatica*. Morphogenesis within the snail proceeds sequentially from the miracidium to the sporocyst, then the redia stage. Each new stage signals an increase in the number of individual immature flukes.

5c    Each redia gives rise to many cercariae, which then penetrate out of the snail and into the water.

6a    The cercariae encyst upon watercress and other littoral plants.

6b    The encysted cercariae, now termed metacercariae, are resistant to mild changes in temperature and some chemicals. The metacercaria is the infective stage of the infection.

7    Sheep are the most commonly infected mammalian hosts in nature, and serve as reservoirs for the human infection. Other herbivores, such as cattle, can also become infected in endemic areas. Experimentally, *F. hepatica* will infect a wide variety of mammals, including the rat and rabbit.

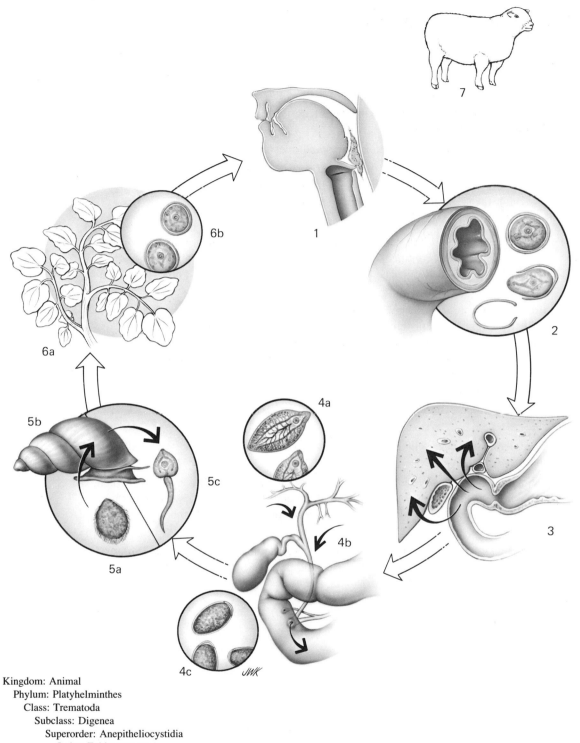

6b

6a

5b

5c

5a

4a

4b

4c

JWK

1

2

3

7

Kingdom: Animal
  Phylum: Platyhelminthes
    Class: Trematoda
      Subclass: Digenea
        Superorder: Anepitheliocystidia
          Order: Echinostomata
            Superfamily: Echinostomatoidea
              Family: Fasciolidae
                Genus: *Fasciola*
                  Species: *hepatica*

# Fasciolopsis Buski

1a  The metacercaria is the infective stage for the human host.

1b  Infection is acquired by swallowing the metacercariae, which have encysted upon freshwater aquatic plants.

2  Excystation occurs in the lumen of the small intestine.

3a  The immature fluke attaches to the luminal surface of the small intestine and begins grazing upon the columnar epithelium of the villus tissue. Maturation to a reproductive adult takes place within 3 months after hatching.

3b  The adult worm measures 25–80 mm in length and 10–20 mm in width.

4  Unembryonated eggs are passed into the lumen of the small intestine and must reach fresh water to continue the life cycle. Each egg measures about 130 μm in length by 75 μm in width, and possesses a terminal operculum. The egg contains the yolk material and a single embryonic cell.

5a  Embryonation proceeds slowly, with the miracidium taking up to 6–8 weeks to fully develop. Hatching ensues, and the ciliated miracidium then seeks out its appropriate intermediate snail host. Upon contact, the miracidium penetrates the snail tissue, develops to the sporocyst stage and migrates to the hepatopancreas. Each sporocyst produces many primary rediae, each of which in turn gives rise to secondary rediae.

5b  The most common genus of snail that serves as the first intermediate host is *Segmentina*.

5c  The secondary rediae give rise to many cercariae, which leave the snail and enter the water.

6  Cercariae of *F. buski* encyst upon a variety of aquatic plants, many of which serve as food for human consumption. Water caltrop (illustrated), water chestnut, and bamboo shoots are among the most common sources of plants upon which encystment occurs.

7  Many mammals besides the human host can also become infected with *Fasciolopsis buski*. Farm animals such as the pig, cat, and dog serve as reservoir hosts.

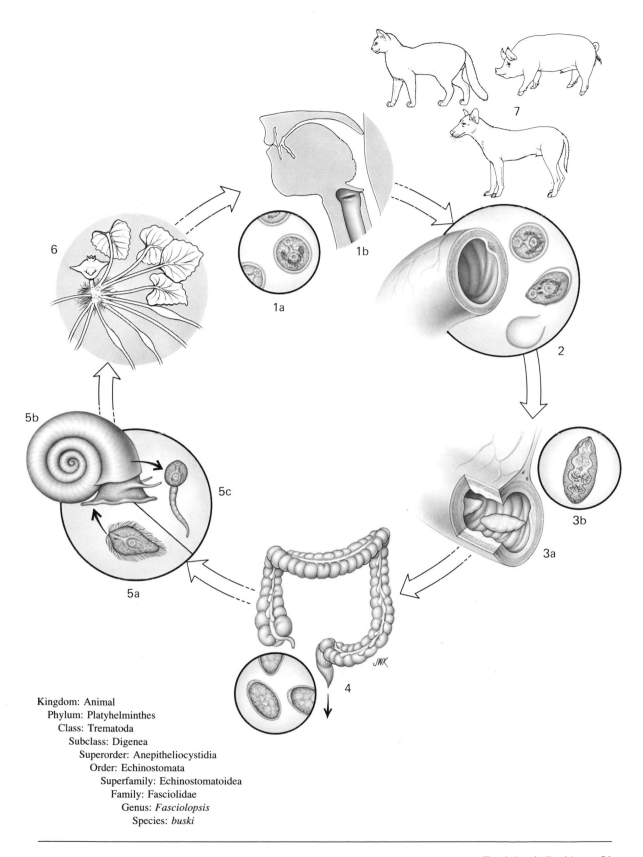

Kingdom: Animal
  Phylum: Platyhelminthes
    Class: Trematoda
      Subclass: Digenea
        Superorder: Anepitheliocystidia
          Order: Echinostomata
            Superfamily: Echinostomatoidea
              Family: Fasciolidae
                Genus: *Fasciolopsis*
                  Species: *buski*

# Paragonimus Westermani

1a  The metacercaria is the infective stage for the human host.

1b  Infection is acquired by ingestion of the metacercaria.

2  The metacercaria excysts within the lumen of the small intestine.

3a  The immature fluke penetrates the small intestine and the diaphragm and migrates into the pleural cavity. There, the worm penetrates lung tissue and takes up residence. Other tissues of the body can also harbor adult worms, such as brain or even striated skeletal muscle. However, these aberrant sites do not lead to completion of the life cycle, since eggs are unable to exit from the body in these locations.

3b  *P. westermani* matures in 8 to 12 weeks after entering the host. The adults usually live as pairs of worms within the necrotic capsule they create while feeding upon lung tissue. Each adult measures 8 to 15 mm long by 5 mm in width. Cross-fertilization is necessary for viable egg production.

4a  Unembryonated eggs are laid in the worm-induced capsule of the lung and pass into the bronchioles.

4b  The unembryonated egg of *P. westermani* measures about 100 μm in length by 55 μm in width, and has a single operculum.

5  Eggs reach fresh water by either being coughed up and expectorated or swallowed and defecated.

6a  The eggs embryonate in fresh water and take 2–3 weeks to fully develop. Hatching ensues, and the ciliated miracidium then swims about seeking its appropriate snail intermediate host. Upon contact, the miracidium penetrates the snail's soft tissue and develops through the sporocyst and redia stages, increasing in numbers during the process.

6b  Snails of the genus *Semisulcospira* are the most common intermediate hosts for *P. westermani*.

6c  Rediae give rise to many cercariae, which, upon leaving the infected snail, swim about until they encounter crustacea.

6d  Freshwater crabs (illustrated) or crayfish are suitable hosts for encystment of the cercariae. The crustacean is penetrated by the cercaria, then the cercaria encysts, transforming into the metacercaria. This is the infective stage for the mammalian host.

7  Besides humans, pigs, dogs, and a wide variety of felines can also harbor the adult of *P. westermani*. Hence there are many potential reservoir hosts for the human infection.

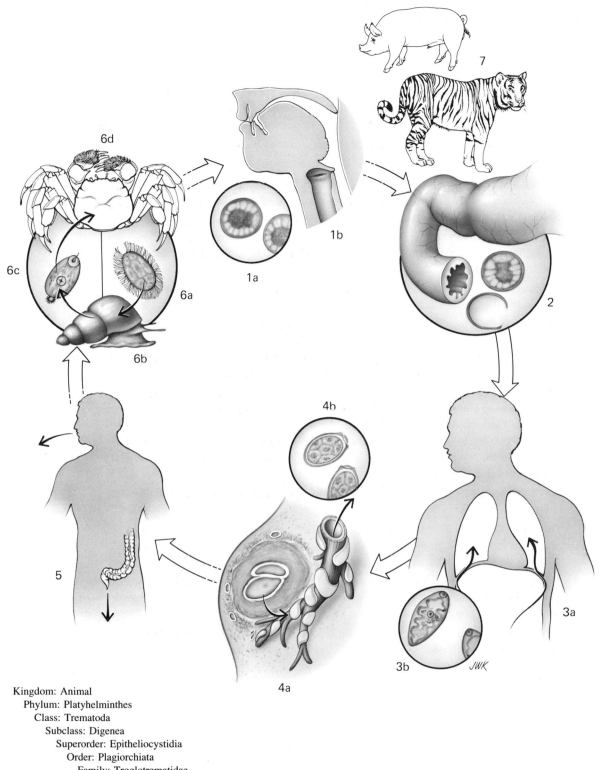

6d

1b

7

6c

6a

1a

6b

2

4h

5

4a

3a

3b

*JWK*

Kingdom: Animal
Phylum: Platyhelminthes
Class: Trematoda
Subclass: Digenea
Superorder: Epitheliocystidia
Order: Plagiorchiata
Family: Troglotrematidae
Genus: *Paragonimus*
Species: *westermani*

# Clonorchis Sinensis

1a    The metacercaria of *Clonorchis sinensis* is the infective stage for the human host.

1b    The metacercaria initiates infection upon ingestion. This occurs when raw or under-cooked infected fish is eaten.

2    The metacercaria excysts in the lumen of the small intestine.

3a    The immature fluke then seeks out its niche in the host.

3b    The immature fluke migrates into the common bile duct and up the biliary tract, completing its growth and development within one of the bile ducts or the gall bladder. Egg production begins about 1 month after infection.

4a    The adult of *Clonorchis sinensis* measures 10–20 mm in length by 2–5 mm in width, and is hermaphroditic. Its food consists of epithelial cells that line the common duct and gallbladder.

4b    The worm releases embryonated eggs which must pass into the lumen of the small intestine if the life cycle is to continue.

4c    The egg of *Clonorchis sinensis* is small compared to the eggs of most other flukes that infect the human host, measuring only 25–30 µm in length by 15 µm in width. It possesses an operculum at one end and a small knoblike protuberance at the other end. Each egg contains a well-developed miracidium.

5a    The egg exits from the host in the feces during defecation and must be deposited in fresh water. Hatching occurs when an appropriate intermediate snail host ingests the eggs. The miracidium then penetrates the wall of the snail's intestine and begins its development within the hepatopancreas. The sporocyst stage is produced first, which, in turn, gives rise to rediae. Each redia produces about 25 cercariae. The entire process takes about 30 days.

5b    Snails in the genus *Parafossarulus* are the most commonly occurring intermediate hosts for *Clonorchis sinensis*.

5c    The cercariae leave the snail and swim about, encysting upon any of a wide variety of freshwater fishes in the family Cyprinidae. Crustaceans can also be infected with the metacercaria of this fluke, but this occurs more rarely than in fish.

5d    When a fish is encountered by a cercaria, the cercaria penetrates beneath the scales of the fish and encysts, transforming into the metacercaria, the infectious stage for the mammalian host.

6    Dogs and cats can also be infected with this fluke, and serve as reservoir hosts for the human infection.

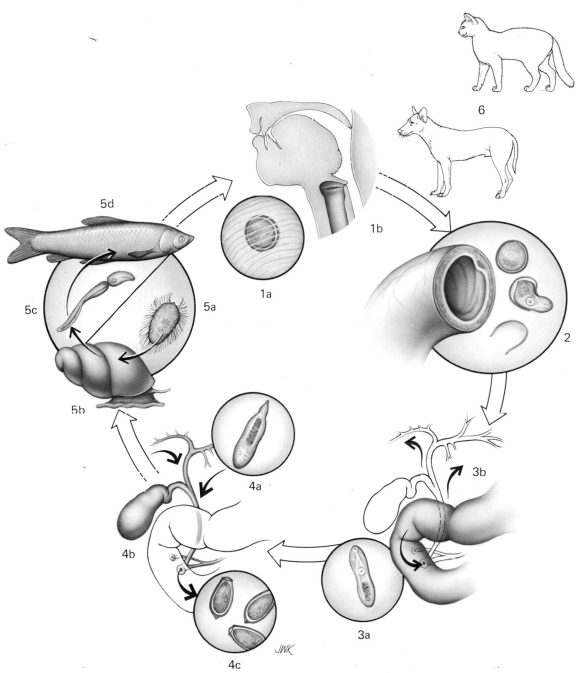

5d

5c

5a

5b

1a

1b

6

2

3b

3a

4a

4b

4c

JWK

Kingdom: Animal
Phylum: Platyhelminthes
Class: Trematoda
Subclass: Digenea
Superorder: Epitheliocystidia
Order: Opisthorchiata
Superfamily: Opisthorchioidea
Family: Opisthorchiidae
Genus: *Clonorchis*
Species: *sinensis*

# Opisthorchis Viverrini

1a Infection in the human host is initiated by the metacercaria.

1b The metacercaria must be ingested; this occurs when raw or undercooked infected fish is eaten.

2  The metacercaria excysts within the lumen of the small intestine.

3a The immature fluke seeks out its niche.

3b After migrating up the biliary tract, the worm feeds upon the epithelium of the bile ducts and develops to an adult worm there.

4a The adult worm is very similar in morphology and size to that of *Clonorchis sinensis*.

4b Eggs must pass out of the bile duct into the lumen of the small intestine in order to continue the life cycle.

4c The egg resembles that of *C. sinensis*.

5a Eggs eventually pass from the host in the feces during defecation. They must then be eaten by an appropriate intermediate snail host. Hatching occurs within the gut tract of the snail. The miracidium burrows into the hepatopancreas and develops into a sporocyst, which produces rediae, which in turn give rise to cercariae.

5b Snails in the genus *Bulinus* are common intermediate hosts for this parasite.

5c The cercariae leave the snail and swim about, seeking a freshwater fish. The cercaria penetrates the fleshy part of the scale and encysts, transforming into the metacercaria.

5d Fish in the family Cyprinidae (e.g., grass carp) serve as important paratenic (i.e., transport) hosts for *O. viverrini*.

6  Dogs, cats, and pigs serve as reservoir hosts for *O. viverrini*.

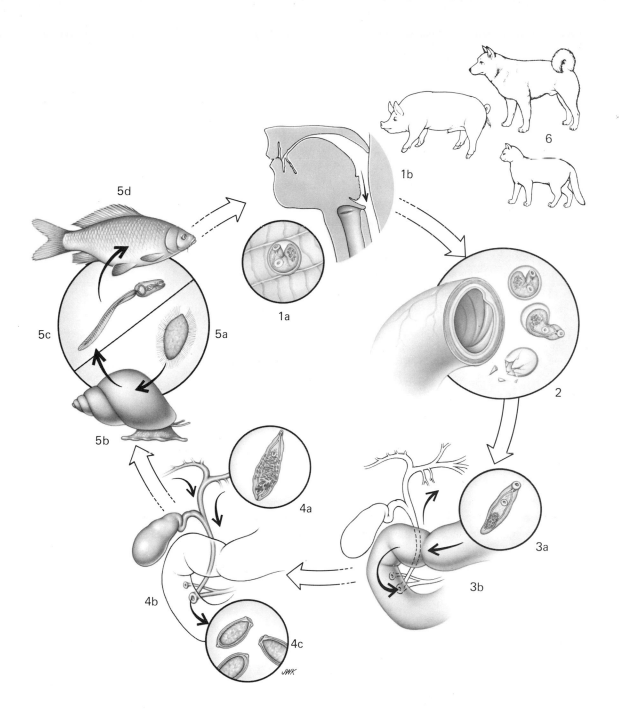

5d

5c

5a

5b

1a

1b

6

2

3a

3b

4a

4b

4c

*JWK*

Kingdom: Animal
  Class: Trematoda
    Subclass: Digenea
      Superorder: Epitheliocystidia
       Order: Opisthorchiata
        Superfamily: Opistohorchioidea
         Family: Opisthorchiidae
          Genus: *Opisthorchis*
           Species: *viverrini*

# Heterophyes Heterophyes

1a  The metacercaria is the infective stage for the mammalian host.

1b  Infection occurs by the oral route when the metacercaria is eaten together with infected raw or undercooked fish.

2  Excystation occurs in the lumen of the small intestine.

3a  The immature fluke attaches to the intestinal villus tissue and proceeds to feed upon epithelial cells. The worm develops to an adult within 8 days after beginning its life in the small intestine.

3b  Each adult worm is 1–2 mm in length by 0.4 mm in width, making it one of the smallest trematodes to infect the human host.

4a  Embryonated eggs are passed directly into the lumen of the small intestine and leave the host during defecation. They must be deposited in fresh water if the life cycle is to continue.

4b  The egg measures 30 μm long by 15 μm wide, and possesses an operculum at one end. Each egg contains a single fully-developed miracidium.

5a  The egg must be ingested by an appropriate intermediate snail host in order to continue the life cycle.

5b  Snails in the genus *Cerithidia* (illustrated) are common hosts in Asia, while those in the genus *Pironella* are important hosts in the Middle East. The miracidium hatches from the egg and penetrates the gut tract of the snail. Development to the sporocyst stage occurs within the hepatopancreas. The sporocyst gives rise to rediae. Many cercariae are produced by each redia.

5c  The cercaria leaves the snail and swims about seeking to encyst upon a fresh- or brackish-water fish. The cercaria, upon coming into contact with the fish, encysts beneath the scales and transforms into the metacercaria, the infectious stage for the mammalian host.

5d  Mullet are the dominant fish upon which *H. heterophyes* encysts.

6  The cat and dog can serve as reservoir hosts for *H. heterophyes*.

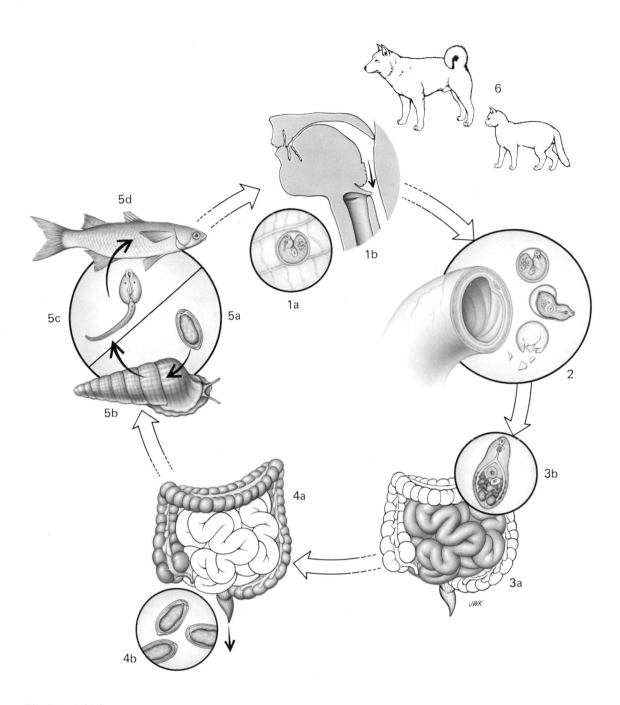

Kingdom: Animal
  Phylum: Platyhelminthes
    Class: Trematoda
      Subclass: Digenea
        Superorder: Epitheliocystidia
          Order: Opisthorchiata
            Superfamily: Opisthorchioidea
              Family: Heterophyidae
                Genus: *Heterophyes*
                  Species: *heterophyes*

# Metagonimus Yokogawai

1a  The infective stage for the mammalian host is the metacercaria. Many fish-eating mammals, in addition to humans, can be infected with *M. yokogawai*.

1b  Infection occurs through the oral route by ingestion of raw or undercooked fish harboring the metacercarial stage.

2   Excystation occurs in the small intestine.

3a  The immature fluke attaches to the villus surface of the small intestine and begins feeding upon epithelium. Development to the adult stage occurs within 10 days after being ingested.

3b  The adult worm measures 1.5 mm long by 0.7 mm wide and lives attached to the wall of the small intestine.

4a  Embryonated eggs are passed into the lumen of the small intestine where they become included within the fecal mass and eventually pass from the host during defecation.

4b  Each egg measures 25 μm long by 15 μm wide and has an operculum. The opposite end is smooth. This egg closely resembles that of *H. heterophyes*. Each egg contains a fully developed miracidium.

5a  Eggs must reach fresh water, where they become ingested by an appropriate intermediate snail host.

5b  Snails in the genus *Semisulcospira* are most frequently infected with *M. yokogawai*. After ingestion, hatching ensues, and the miracidium penetrates the gut tract and begins its development in the hepatopancreas. The miracidium transforms into the sporocyst stage, which, in turn, gives rise to the redia stage. Numerous cercariae are produced by each redia.

5c  The cercaria penetrates out of the snail and swims about, seeking a freshwater fish. When a cercaria encounters a fish, it penetrates beneath scale and encysts, transforming into the metacercaria, the infectious stage for the mammalian host.

5d  Fish in the genus *Plecoglossus* are commonly infected with metacercaria of *M. yokogawai*.

6   The dog and cat are the most common reservoir hosts for *M. yokogawai*.

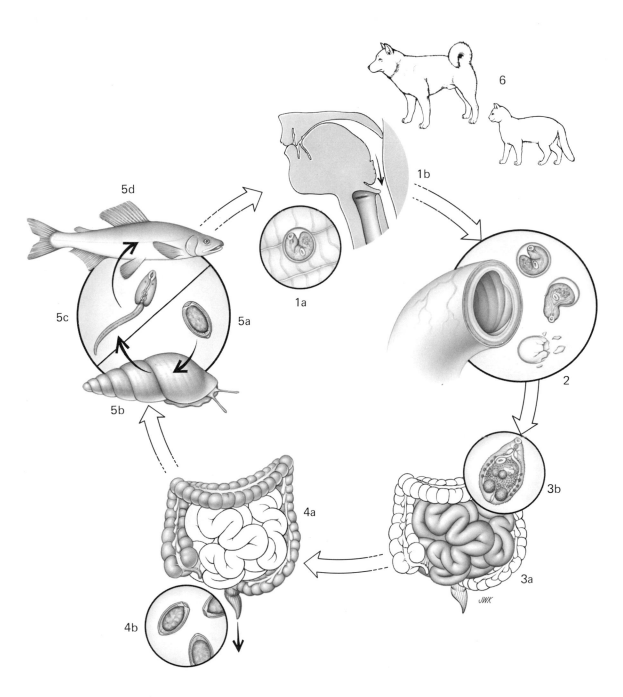

5d

5c

5a

5b

1a

1b

6

2

3b

3a

JWK

4a

4b

Kingdom: Animal
  Phylum: Platyhelminthes
    Class: Trematoda
      Subclass: Digenea
        Superorder: Epitheliocystidia
          Order: Opisthorchiata
            Superfamily: Opisthorchioidea
              Family: Heterophyidae
                Genus: *Metagonimus*
                  Species: *yokogawai*

# 4 Nematoda

# General Characteristics of Nematodes

Nematodes comprise a large group of organisms, the majority of which are free-living. Characteristically, they are nonsegmented round worms, and the sexes are separate and usually morphologically distinct. The life cycles of parasitic nematodes can be rather simple. For example, some species of nematodes lay eggs that leave the host in feces and embryonate in soil. In these cases, the eggs enter the host by the oral route and the worms develop to adults in the intestinal tract. Other species of nematodes have more complex cycles, involving intermediate invertebrate or vertebrate hosts, often with complex migration routes, once inside the host. The route of entry into the host can also vary, with some species being capable of penetrating directly into the host through the unbroken skin. Nematode parasites have been selected for life in a broad spectrum of niches within the mammalian host, including intracellular and intramulticellular environments.

Structurally, all nematodes are similar, being covered by a thick, acellular collagen-rich cuticle. A hypodermal region directly beneath the cuticle synthesizes new cuticula before each molt, and also serves as a point of attachment for muscles. All nematodes molt four times as larvae before developing to adulthood. With each molt, the worm achieves a more advanced stage of development. All muscle cells contain both thick and thin filaments and, uniquely, insert processes into the lateral, dorsal, and ventral nerve branches, which run the length of the worm. Adult worms possess a complete gut tract, typically subdivided into three regions; namely, foregut (pharynx and esophagus), midgut, and hindgut. The foregut and hindgut are lined with an extension of the outer cuticle, while the epithelium of the midgut is covered with microvilli and usually serves as the absorption surface through which nutrients enter the pseudocoelom. For many species, the source of food is known. For example, *Ascaris lumbricoides* adults ingest whatever food the host has eaten, while hookworm adults feed directly on villous tissue and, in addition, suck blood. In contrast, for *Trichinella spiralis* and *Trichuris trichiura,* the food sources remain unknown.

Metabolically, parasitic nematodes possess both aerobic and anaerobic energy pathways, and complete metabolic pathways for synthesizing all classes of macromolecules.

The nervous system consists of an anterior nerve ring from which emanate the dorsal, ventral, and lateral branches. A number of sensory nerve endings are found clustered near the anterior and/or posterior ends of the adult stage of most species of round worms. These aid the nematode in navigating through the many microenvironments of the host, and also enable male and female worms to find each other in the milieu of the host prior to mating.

The excretory system consists of two lateral tubes and associated anterior pores. A large portion of worm biomass is devoted to reproduction. The female reproductive tract is tubelike and consists of the ovary, seminal receptacle, uterus, oviduct, and vulva. Many species lay eggs, while others give birth to live larvae. The male reproductive tract consists of the testis, seminal vesicle, vas deferens, and cloaca. Sperm are nonflagellated amoeboidlike cells, which are deposited into the vulval opening during copulation.

# Classification

**Bold type** indicates families represented in book by parasites

Phylum: Nematoda
  Class: Aphasmida
    Order: Trichurata
      Family: Anatrichosomatidae
      **Family: Capillariidae**
      Family: Cystoopsidae
      **Family: Trichinellidae**
      Family: Trichosomoididae
      **Family: Trichuridae**
    Order: Dioctophymata
      Family: Dioctophymatidae
      Family: Eustrongylidae
      Family: Soboliphymatidae
  Class: Phasmidea
    Order: Rhabditata
      Family: Rhabdiasidae
      **Family: Strongyloididae**
    Order: Strongylata
      Family: Amidostomatidae
      **Family: Ancylostomatidae**
      Family: Angiostrongylidae
      Family: Cloacinidae
      Family: Cyathostomidae
      Family: Deletrocephalidae
      Family: Diaphanocephalidae
      Family: Dictyocaulidae
      Family: Filaroididae
      Family: Heligmosomatidae
      Family: Ichthyostrongylidae
      Family: Metastrongylidae
      Family: Oesophagostomatidae
      Family: Ollulanidae
      Family: Pharyngostrongylidae
      Family: Protostrongylidae
      Family: Pseudaliidae
      Family: Stephanuridae
      Family: Strongylacanthidae
      Family: Strongylidae
      Family: Syngamidae
      Family: Trichostrongylidae
    Order: Ascaridata
      Family: Acanthocheilidae

Family: Angusticaecidae
Family: Anisakidae
**Family: Ascaridae**
Family: Ascaridiidae
Family: Crossophoridae
Family: Goeziidae
Family: Heterocheilidae
Family: Inglisonematidae
Family: Oxyascarididae
**Family: Toxocaridae**
  Order: Oxyurata
    Superfamily: Oxyuroidea
      Family: Heteroxynematidae
      **Family: Oxyuridae**
      Family: Ozolamidae
      Family: Pharyngodonidae
      Family: Syphaciidae
    Superfamily: Atractoidea
      Family: Atractidae
      Family: Crossocephalidae
      Family: Cruziidae
      Family: Hoplodontophoridae
      Family: Labiduridae
      Family: Schrankianidae
      Family: Travnematidae
    Superfamily: Cosmocercoidea
      Family: Cosmocercidae
      Family: Gyrinicolidae
      Family: Lauroiidae
    Superfamily: Heterakoidea
      Family: Aspidoderidae
      Family: Heterakidae
      Family: Spinicaudidae
      Family: Strongyluridae
    Superfamily: Kathlaniodea
      Family: Kathlaniidae
    Superfamily: Subuluroidea
      Family: Maupasinidae
      Family: Parasubuluridae
      Family: Subuluridae
  Order: Spirurata
    Family: Acuariidae

Family: Ascaropsidae
Family: Cobboldinidae
Family: Crassicaudidae
Family: Desmidocercidae
Family: Gnathostomatidae
Family: Gongylonematidae
Family: Habronematidae
Family: Haplonematidae
Family: Hedruidae
Family: Physalopteridae
Family: Pneumospiruridae
Family: Rhabdochonidae
Family: Rictulariidae
Family: Salobrellidae
Family: Schistorophidae
Family: Seuratidae
Family: Spinitectidae
Family: Spirocercidae
Family: Spiruridae
Family: Streptocaridae
Family: Tetrameridae
Family: Thelaziidae
  Order: Camallanata
    Family: Anguillicodidae
    Family: Camallanidae
    **Family: Dracunculidae**
    Family: Oceanicucullanidae
    Family: Philometridae
    Family: Phlyctainophoridae
    Family: Skrjabillanidae
    Family: Tetanonematidae
  Order: Filariata
    Family: Aproctidae
    Family: Desmidocercidae
    Family: Diplotriaenidae
    Family: Filariidae
    **Family: Onchocercidae**
    Family: Setariidae

# Capillaria Philippinensis

1a  The third stage larva is the infectious stage of *Capillaria philippinensis*.

1b  Infection is initiated by ingestion of certain species of uncooked fresh or brackish water fish and crustaceans which are infected with third-stage larvae.

2  Larvae are released from the intermediate host tissue in the stomach. They then are carried to the small intestine where they penetrate into the villous tissue and develop into adults. The adult female measures 3–5 mm in length and 30 $\mu$m in diameter, while the male measures 1–2 mm in length and 30 $\mu$m in diameter.

3a  Adult females begin their reproductive cycle by shedding first-stage larvae.

3b  These larvae are capable of infecting the same host by penetrating adjacent villous tissue, molting four times, and developing into adults. Thus large numbers of worms can accumulate in the small intestinal tissue in a few weeks.

3c  Within weeks after infection, adult females switch to egg production. What factors control this change in reproductive strategy are not yet known.

3d  The eggs reach the lumen of the small intestine.

4  Fertilized eggs exit from the host in the feces.

5a-c  In order for the cycle to continue, eggs (5a) must reach fresh or brackish water where they complete their embryonation. They are ingested by small fish (5b) and crustaceans (5c). Little is known about the infection in the intermediate host. Experimental infection in various water birds has been successfully carried out. Thus, birds may be capable of serving as reservoir hosts.

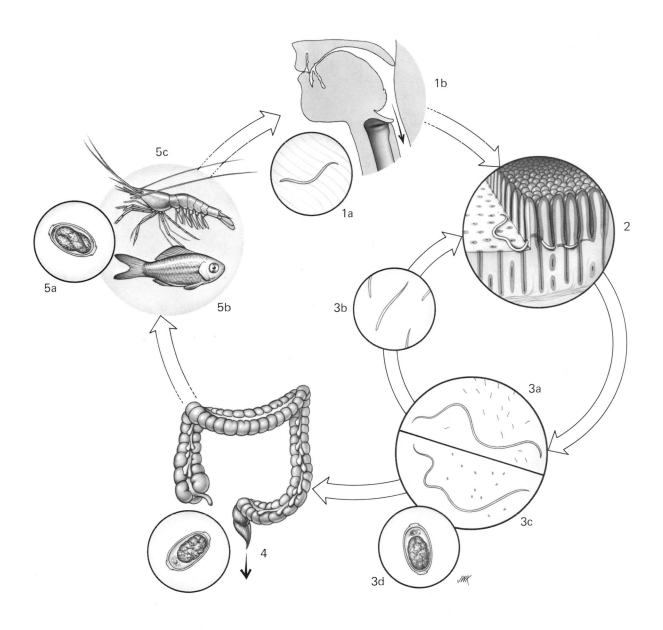

1b
5c
1a
2
5a
3b
5b
3a
4
3c
3d
JWK

Kingdom: Animal
　Phylum: Nematoda
　　Class: Aphasmida
　　　Order: Trichurata
　　　　Family: Capillariidae
　　　　　Genus: *Capillaria*
　　　　　　Species: *philippinensis*

# Trichinella Spiralis

## Enteral Phase

1  *Trichinella spiralis* is not host specific. All mammals are susceptible. Infection begins by the ingestion of infected raw or undercooked unfrozen meat containing the infectious first-stage larvae in striated skeletal muscle tissue. At this point the worm is 1 mm in length by 35 μm in diameter.

2  Parasites are freed of host tissue by digestive enzymes in the stomach and then are delivered to the small intestine.

3  Within the small intestine the larva quickly penetrates a row of columnar epithelium. It is now considered an intramulticellular parasite. There, the worm undergoes four molts within 28 hours, developing into an adult male or female.

4  Mating occurs within 30 hours after infection. The precise location in the gut where mating takes place is still undetermined. After mating (shown here in cross section) adult worms reside within the intramulticellular niche.

5a  Males are 1.5 mm by 36 μm, while females (shown here) are 3 mm in length by 36 μm in diameter.

5b  Within 5–6 days following infection, females begin shedding newborn (first-stage) larvae into the intracellular milieu. Newborn larvae are 80 μm in length by 6–7 μm in diameter. The newborn larva penetrates through the villous tissue into the lamina propria by using a spearlike stylet within its esophagus. They then enter either a draining lymph or blood vessel.

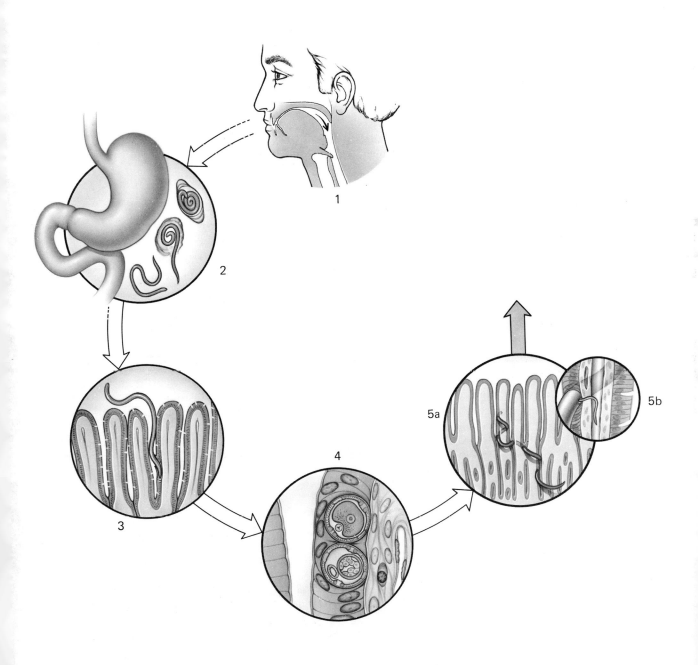

Kingdom: Animal
Phylum: Nematoda
Class: Aphasmida
Order: Trichurata
Family: Trichinellidae
Genus: *Trichinella*
Species: *spiralis*

# Trichinella Spiralis

## Parenteral Phase

6    Larvae eventually enter the general circulation and become distributed throughout the body.

7a    Penetration of tissue by newborn larvae appears to occur solely by use of its esophageal stylet.

7b    Migrating newborns penetrate out of capillaries into whatever tissue happens to be adjacent to the vessel, but will only remain within striated skeletal muscle cells. Larvae in tissues other than muscle reenter the general circulation.

8    The larvae grow and differentiate within the intracellular matrix of the infected muscle cell. During the process, the larva induces dramatic changes in the muscle cell, resulting in a totally new arrangement of host cytoplasm. Most of the cellular changes are complete by day 9 after intracellular infection.

9    Further host cell modifications at day 10–12 result in a nearly mature unit now referred to as the Nurse cell. The name describes the activity of this cell, the purpose of which is to facilitate nutrient acquisition by the larva and export of its metabolic wastes.

10    The larva-Nurse cell complex is fully grown at day 20 after infection. The first-stage larva has now achieved its maximum growth.

11    Any species of mammal can serve as a reservoir host for the infection, but transmission from animal to animal is largely by carnivorism and scavenging. In most of Europe, Asia and North America the pig is the usual source of infection. Polar bears, wart hogs and bush pigs are reservoirs commonly responsible for infections in arctic and tropical environments.

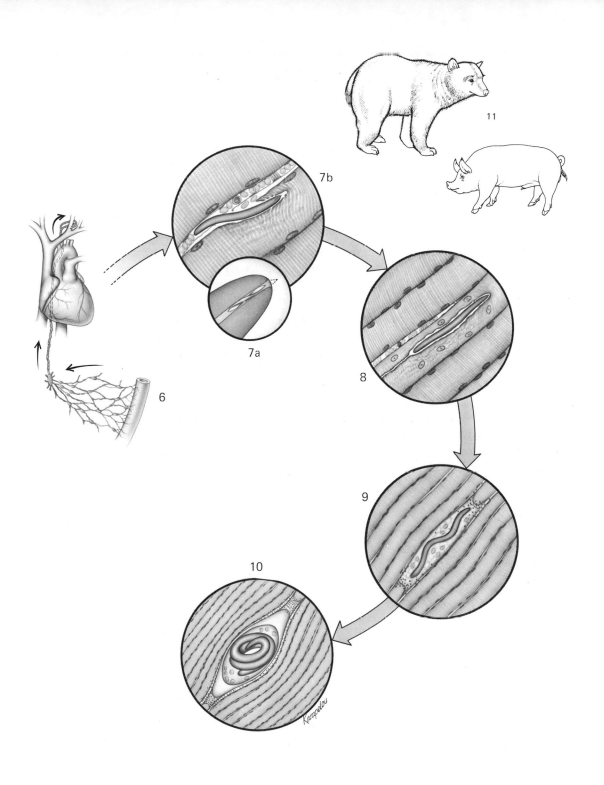

# Trichuris Trichiura (Whipworm)

1 Infection with *Trichuris trichiura* is initiated by ingestion of embryonated eggs. Feces-contaminated soil and various uncooked vegetables that have been fertilized with human feces are the two most common sources of such eggs. Because of their impervious outer shell, embryonated eggs can survive in warm, moist soil for many months to years without losing their infectivity.

2 The egg contains a first-stage larva, which hatches upon reaching the small intestine.

3 Peristalsis carries the larvae to the large intestine, where they penetrate into the epithelium. After four molts, the worms, now adults, copulate. The female measures 4–6 cm in length and 1–2 mm in width at its thickest point. The male is somewhat smaller, measuring 2–3 cm in length and 0.6–0.8 mm in width.

4 The anterior portion of each worm remains embedded in a parasite-induced host syncytium composed of fused epithelial cells, while the posterior portion of the worm protrudes into the lumen of the large intestine. Worms begin producing eggs about 1 to 1½ months after infection. Female worms shed about 3,000–5,000 fertilized unembryonated eggs each day, and may continue to do so for up to 2 years.

5 Eggs must be deposited in a suitable external environment for development to continue. Loamy, warm, moist soil represents an ideal niche for embryonation. Larvae are fully developed into first-stage worms within 2–3 weeks after deposition. The entire life cycle, from egg to adult to egg takes approximately 2 months. There are no reservoir hosts for infection with *Trichuris trichiura*.

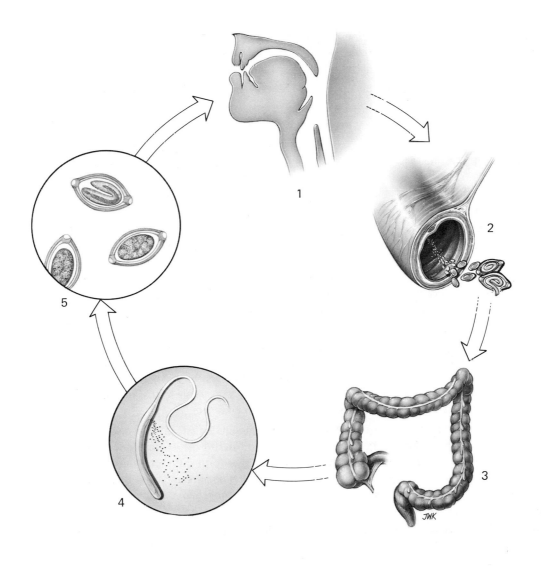

1

2

5

4

3

JWK

Kingdom: Animal
 Phylum: Nematoda
  Class: Aphasmida
   Order: Trichurata
    Family: Trichuridae
     Genus: *Trichuris*
      Species: *trichiura*

# Strongyloides Stercoralis

1  The third-stage (filariform) infectious larva enters the host by penetrating the unbroken skin. Infection can also occur by ingestion of this stage. The larva penetrates into a capillary and is carried passively into the general circulation.

2  Larvae reach the pulmonary circulation where they penetrate out of the alveolar capillaries into the alveolar spaces.

3  Larvae migrate up the respiratory tree into the pharynx and are then swallowed.

4  *S. stercoralis* parasitic larvae develop only to adult females within the villus tissue of the small intestine. Male worms only exist in the free-living cycle. Reproduction in the parasitic female is by a process involving sequential production of sperm, then eggs. She is a protanderous hermaphrodite, measuring 2 mm in length by 0.04 mm in width.

5  Within several weeks after developing to adulthood, the worms begin to shed fully embryonated eggs into the surrounding tissue. There, the embryos develop to first-, then to second-stage larvae, after which they hatch. Once free of the eggshell, the second-stage larvae migrate out into the lumen of the small intestine. The worms are carried passively to the large intestine, where they are included within the fecal mass, and are defecated into the external environment.

6  If feces containing larvae are deposited in warm, moist, loamy or sandy soil, then the larvae feed, grow, and molt twice more, developing into free-living males and females. Several reproductive cycles can occur in this situation, provided that moisture, temperature, and food remain optimal. Many infectious third-stage larvae can result from the free-living cycle. Thus, the soil serves as a reservoir for the infection. The entire free-living life cycle takes several weeks to complete.

7  Individuals suffering from any one of a number of immunological difficiencies may permit second-stage larvae to develop into third-stage (filariform) worms within the lumen of the large intestine. When this occurs, the filariform larva can infect the same host by penetrating the large intestine, entering the bloodstream and completing the migration as described here in steps 1–3. Hence, *Strongyloides stercoralis* can be autoinfectious.

8  Many animals can serve as reservoir hosts, including dogs and monkeys.

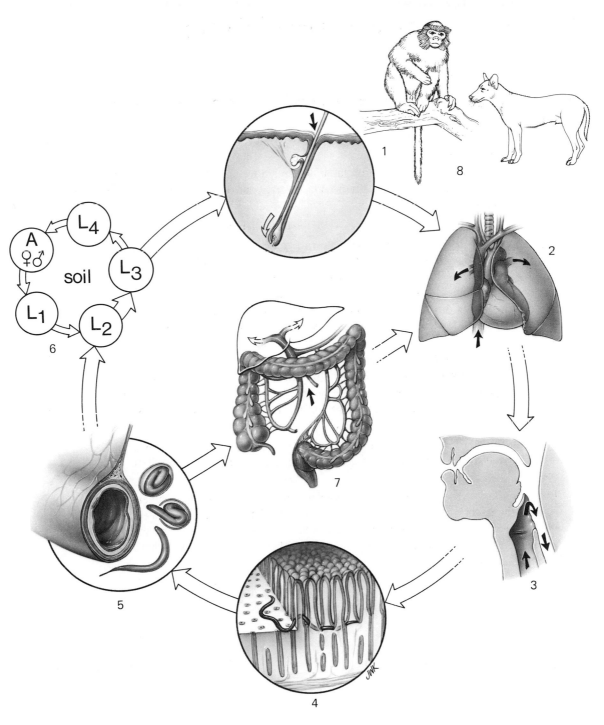

soil

Kingdom: Animal
Phylum: Nematoda
Class: Phasmida
Order: Rhabditata
Family: Strongyloididae
Genus: *Strongyloides*
Species: *stercoralis*

# Necator Americanus (Hookworm)

1a  The infectious filariform (third-stage) larva enters the host by either penetrating the unbroken skin or by being ingested.

1b  Larvae penetrating skin usually enter the circulation through a capillary at the base of a hair shaft.

2   Worms are passively carried through the bloodstream to the heart, where they are pumped into the pulmonary circulation and penetrate out of an alveolar capillary into the alveolar space.

3   After crawling up the respiratory tract to the pharynx, larvae are swallowed.

4   Upon arrival in the lumen of the small intestine, larvae attach to the villous tissue, molt twice, and develop to adults. The female is 10 mm in length by 0.35 mm in width, while the male is 7 mm in length by 0.30 mm in width. Mating ensues with male and female worms living *in copula*. Each female produces about 10,000 eggs each day. Worms live for about 2–4 years. Adult worms feed directly on villous tissue and suck blood. It is not known whether worms use blood as a food source.

5   Eggs are passed fertilized and begin to embryonate immediately. Feces containing eggs must be deposited in warm, moist, sandy or loamy soil if the life cycle is to continue. Embryogenesis is rapid, taking only 3–5 days. The larvae hatch in feces and consume bacteria, developing to rhabditiform (second-stage) larvae, then molt again into filariform (third-stage) worms.

6a  The filariform larvae do not feed, and, as already mentioned, are the infectious stage. The life cycle from larva to adult to filariform larva takes about 1 to 1½ months.

6b  Infectious larvae seek out the highest object in their immediate environment and remain there during periods of maximum moisture. This usually correlates with the early daylight hours. When moisture levels drop, they retreat into the soil and remain there until conditions favor migration. There are no reservoir hosts for *Necator americanus*.

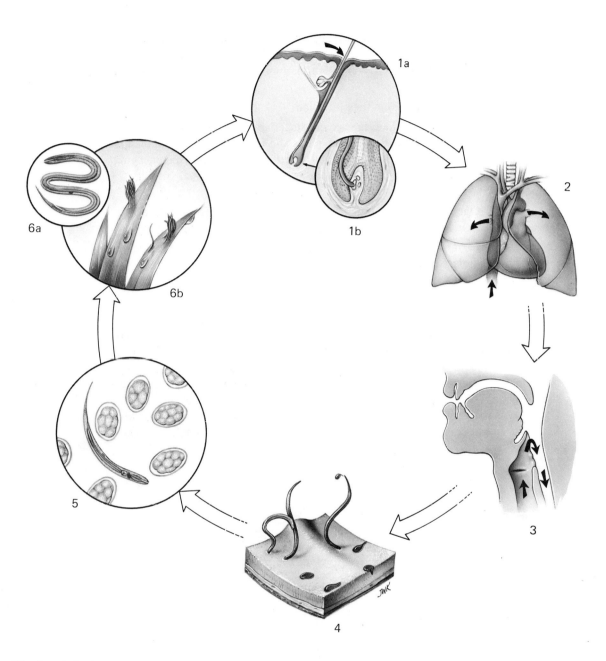

Kingdom: Animal
Phylum: Nematoda
Class: Phasmida
Order: Strongylata
Family: Ancylostomatidae
Genus: *Necator*
Species: *americanus*

# Ascaris Lumbricoides (Giant Intestinal Worm)

1a  The embryonated egg is the infectious stage of *Ascaris lumbricoides*. Feces-contaminated raw vegetables are the most common sources of eggs. Like *Trichuris*, the eggs of *A. lumbricoides* can survive in warm, moist, sandy or loamy soil for months or even years.

1b  Eggs are swallowed in order to initiate infection.

2   Upon reaching the small intestine, the second-stage larva is stimulated to hatch. It then rapidly penetrates the small intestinal villus and enters the portal circulation. It arrives in the liver, and then penetrates out of the capillary into the parenchyma. The larva develops to a third-stage worm during this brief (1–2 weeks) migratory period.

3   The third-stage larva is now larger in diameter than a capillary. The worm reenters the returning circulation to the heart and is pumped into the pulmonary artery.

4   Worms become stuck in the small vessels of the alveolus, where they penetrate out into the alveolar spaces.

5   *A. lumbricoides* larvae migrate up the respiratory tract to the pharynx, and become swallowed.

6   After two more molts in the small intestinal lumen, worms grow to their full length; a process that takes 3 months. The adult female is 20–35 cm in length, by 0.5 cm in diameter, while the male is smaller, measuring 15–20 cm in length by 0.3–0.8 cm in diameter. Ascaris adults ingest and utilize intestinal luminal contents. After mating, the female begins to produce fertilized unembryonated eggs at the rate of about 200,000 per day. *Ascaris* adults can live up to 5 years, but average 2½ to 3 years. Eggs embryonate in soil, and take 2–4 weeks to do so. The entire life cycle from egg to adult to egg takes from 3½ to 4 months to complete. There are no reservoir hosts for Ascaris.

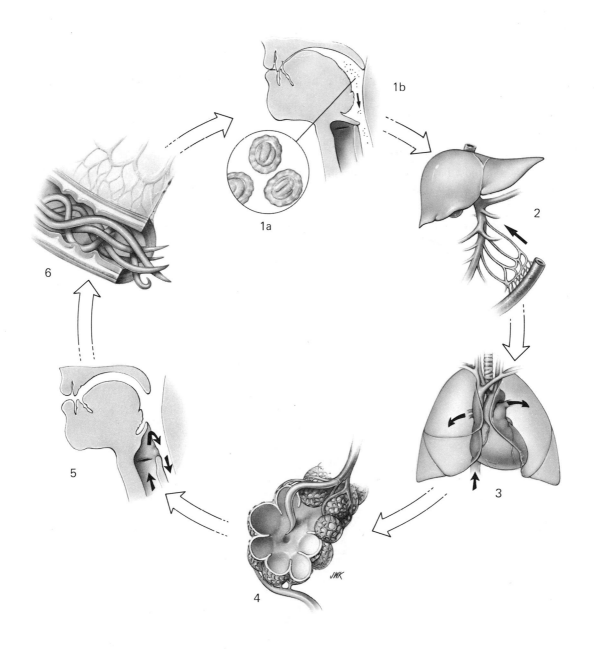

1a

1b

2

3

4

5

6

JWK

Kingdom: Animal
Phylum: Nematoda
Class: Phasmida
Order: Ascaridata
Family: Ascaridae
Genus: *Ascaris*
Species: *lumbricoides*

# Toxocara Canis and Cati

1a  The adults of *Toxocara canis* and *cati* live in the lumen of the small intestine of dogs and cats, respectively.

1b  The life cycle in dogs and cats is similar to that of *Ascaris lumbricoides* in the human host (see pages 110 and 111).

2   In all hosts, infection begins by ingestion of embryonated eggs containing the second stage larva.

3   Larvae hatch in the small intestine.

4   In the human host larvae penetrate the small intestine, enter the portal circulation and wander aimlessly from organ to organ. Parasites develop only to the third larval stage in the human host.

5   Organs most frequently infected include the liver (5a), the brain (5b) and the eye (5c). In contrast its cycle continues in dogs and cats resulting in adult worms in the small intestinal lumen.

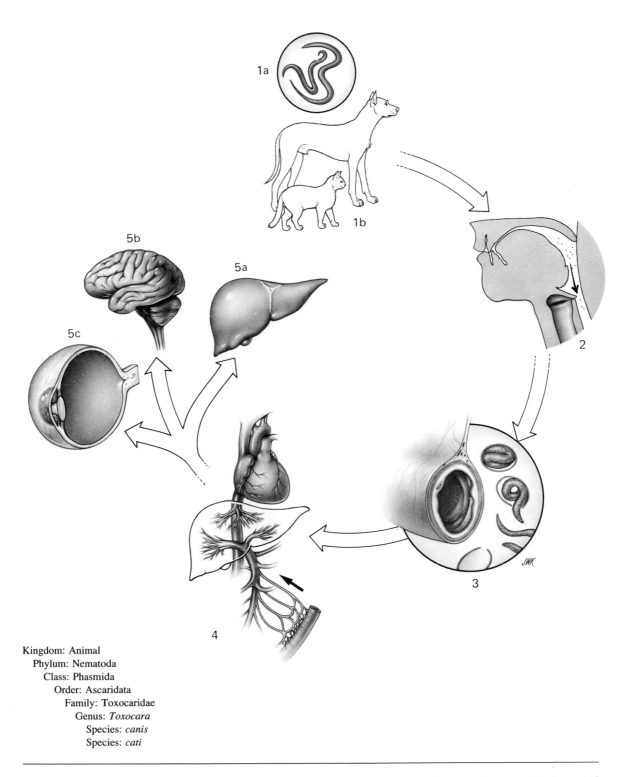

1a

1b

5b

5a

5c

2

3

4

JWK

Kingdom: Animal
    Phylum: Nematoda
        Class: Phasmida
            Order: Ascaridata
                Family: Toxocaridae
                    Genus: *Toxocara*
                        Species: *canis*
                        Species: *cati*

# Enterobius Vermicularis (Pinworm)

1    Infection with *Enterobius vermicularis* is usually initiated by ingestion of embryonated eggs. Eggs can also hatch on the perianal region and infect via the anus. Aberrant infections result from larvae migrating into the vaginal tract instead of the anus.

2    The embryonated egg contains the larva. As it is carried down the small intestine, it develops further and comes to reside in the lumen of the transverse and descending colon as an adult. Male worms measure 0.2 mm in width by 2.5 mm in length, while females measure 0.5 mm in width by 8–13 mm in length.

3    Mating occurs in the colon. Gravid females each contain from 10,000 to 11,000 eggs. The gravid females, in response to lower body temperature, reduced oxygen tension, or both, migrate out of the body, usually while the person is asleep.

4    The female worms come to rest on the area surrounding the anus.

5a    There they either experience prolapse of their uterus, or simply die and disintegrate.

5b    The embryonated eggs develop within 6 hours to first-, then second-stage worms. The larvae are now infectious. The outer egg shell is thin and susceptible to drying. Pinworm larvae die within 2 to 3 days in a low-humidity environment. The entire cycle from egg to adult to egg takes approximately 6 weeks.

6    Repeated infections eventually sensitize the host to worm antigens. The resulting itching and scratching cycle facilitates the contamination of fingers with embryonated eggs, which in turn ensures the reinfection of the same host. There are no reservoir hosts for this parasite. Furthermore, the human host is not susceptible to infection from any other species of pinworm.

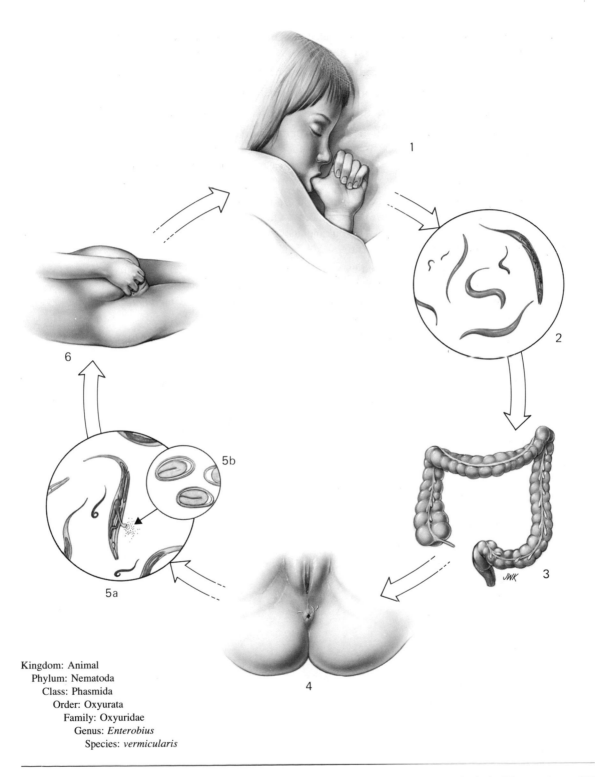

Kingdom: Animal
Phylum: Nematoda
Class: Phasmida
Order: Oxyurata
Family: Oxyuridae
Genus: *Enterobius*
Species: *vermicularis*

# Dracunculus Medinensis

1    Infection begins by drinking water contaminated with microscopic crustaceans (e.g., cyclops) which are infected with the third-stage larvae of *D. medinensis*.

2a    The infected crustaceans are digested in the stomach, freeing the infectious larva.

2b    The worm is carried passively by peristalsis to the small intestine.

3    The larva penetrates the small intestine and enters the subcutaneous tissues.

4    Larvae migrate within this tissue to the lower extremities. Adult males and females develop within the subcutaneous tissues. Females are 100 mm in length by 1.5 mm in width, while the males are much smaller, measuring only 40 mm in length by 0.4 mm in width.

5a    Following mating, the female induces a fluid-filled blister at her anteriormost end. Upon encountering water, the worm experiences a uterine prolapse, releasing live first-stage larvae into the blister fluid. Simultaneously, the blister ruptures, releasing the larvae into the aquatic environment.

5b    The motile larvae are quickly ingested by various species of crustaceans. The worms penetrate into the hemocoel and develop to third-stage infectious larvae within 2–3 weeks. None of the various mammals susceptible to infection with *D. medinensis* are thought to serve as reservoirs of infections for the human host.

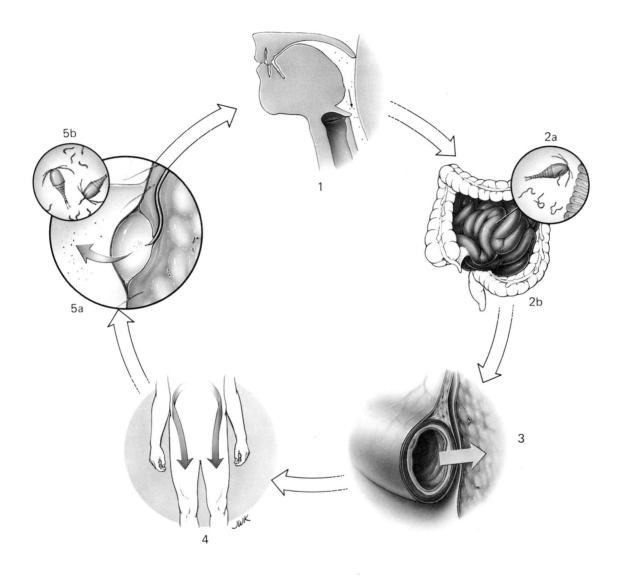

1

2a

2b

3

5b

5a

4

JWK

Kingdom: Animal
Phylum: Nematoda
Class: Phasmida
Order: Camallanata
Family: Dracunculidae
Genus: *Dracunculus*
Species: *medinensis*

# Wuchereria Bancrofti

1a   *Wuchereria bancrofti* is transmitted from person to person by culicine and anopheline mosquitoes.

1b   When an infected mosquito bites, the infectious third-stage larva crawls out of the biting mouthparts of the mosquito onto the skin. When she withdraws her mouthparts after taking a blood meal, the larva crawls into the bite wound.

2   Worms migrate by the lymph to the draining lymph nodes.

3   Adult males and females develop to sexual maturity in the afferent lymph vessels adjacent to the lymph nodes. Females are 8 cm long by 300 $\mu$m in diameter, and males are 4 cm long by 100 $\mu$m in diameter. Development in the mammalian host is slow, taking approximately 1 year to complete.

4   Females give birth to living larvae called microfilariae. These larvae migrate through the lymph node, and eventually enter the general circulation of the blood. Microfilariae are 270 $\mu$m in length by 9 $\mu$m in diameter and live for about 1½ years.

5a   *W. bancrofti,* in most places in the world, exhibits periodic behavior. Microfilariae are found in peripheral blood of those individuals experiencing periods of extended rest (i.e., sleep).

5b   Microfilariae are not found in peripheral blood during periods of physical activity. In some geographic regions, *W. bancrofti* exhibits non-periodic behavior (i.e., they are found in peripheral blood at all times).

6   When a mosquito ingests blood containing microfilariae, the blood is digested, and the worms penetrate the intestine, enter the hemocoel, then migrate to the flight wing muscles in the thorax. There, they penetrate single muscle fibers and grow and develop to third-stage infectious larvae. Following maturation, they migrate into the hemocoel and take up residence in the biting mouthparts. Infectious larvae develop within 2 weeks after being ingested. There are no reservoir hosts for *Wuchereria bancrofti.*

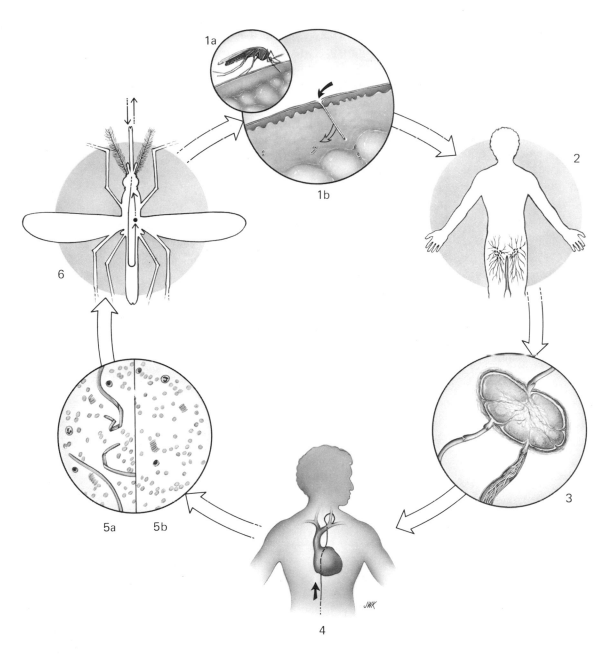

1a
1b
2
3
4
5a  5b
6

Kingdom: Animal
Phylum: Nematoda
Class: Phasmida
Order: Filariata
Family: Onchocercidae
Genus: *Wuchereria*
Species: *bancrofti*

# Loa Loa

1a  Dipteran flies in the genus *Chrysops* are the vectors for *Loa loa*.

1b  Infection occurs when an infected fly takes a blood meal. The third-stage larvae crawl out of the biting mouthparts onto the skin adjacent to the bite site. When the fly leaves the host, the larvae enter the bite wound and migrate to the subcutaneous tissues.

2  Larvae grow to adulthood in the subcutaneous tissues. Adult male and female *L. loa* develop to sexual maturity within 1–4 years after initial infection. Females are 60 mm long by 0.5 mm wide. Males are 32 mm long by 0.4 mm wide. Females give birth to live larvae (microfilariae), which find their way into the general circulation of the blood.

3  Microfilariae exhibit diurnal periodicity, appearing in peripheral blood during daylight hours, and remaining sequestered in the deep vascular beds of the lungs at night.

4  *Chrysops* spp. feed during daylight hours, acquiring their infection by taking a blood meal from an infected individual.

5  The microfilariae penetrate the intestine, enter the hemocoel, and then migrate to the flight wing muscles where they each penetrate a single muscle fiber. After two molts, they are fully infectious. The larvae then migrate out of the muscle tissue into the hemocoel, then into the biting mouthparts. There are no reservoir hosts for this parasite.

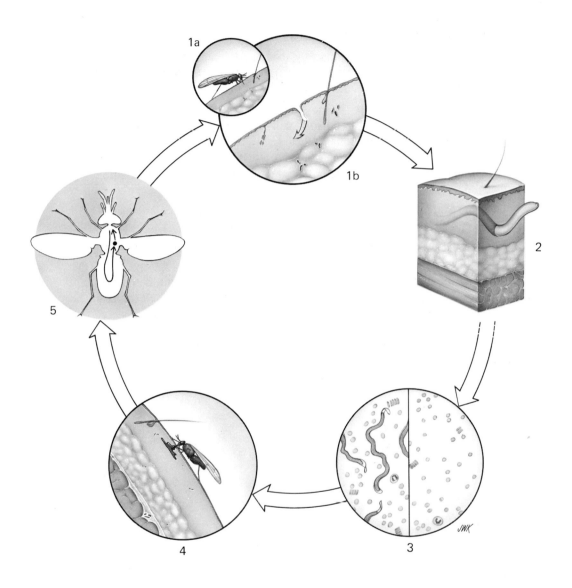

Kingdom: Animal
  Phylum: Nematoda
    Class: Phasmida
      Order: Filariata
        Family: Onchocercidae
          Genus: *Loa*
            Species: *loa*

# Onchocerca Volvulus

1a  The female blackfly (*Simulium* sp.) is the vector of *Onchocerca volvulus*.

1b  The infective larva crawls out of the blackfly mouthparts onto the bite site while the infected insect feeds. When it withdraws its mouthparts, the larva crawls into the wound and enters the subcutaneous tissues.

2  Larvae molt and develop to adults in the subcutaneous tissue within a parasite-induced nodule, and take one year to do so. Adult females are 45–50 cm in length by 300 μm in diameter, while the smaller males are 20–40 mm in length by 200 μm in diameter. After mating, each female begins to shed live larvae (microfilariae). Adult worms can live for 8–10 years and produce hundreds of thousands of offspring during that time.

3  Microfilariae migrate away from the adult worm, remaining within the confines of the subcutaneous tissue. Microfilariae can live for up to 6 months.

4  The larvae are ingested by female blackflies when they take a blood meal from an infected person.

5  Once within the blackfly, the larvae penetrate the intestine, enter the hemocoel, and migrate to the flight wing muscles, where they penetrate into single muscle fibers. Two molts ensue within 6 days, resulting in an infectious (third-stage) larva. The worms then migrate to the mouthparts and are introduced onto the host during the next blood meal that the insect takes. No reservoir hosts exist for *Onchocerca volvulus*.

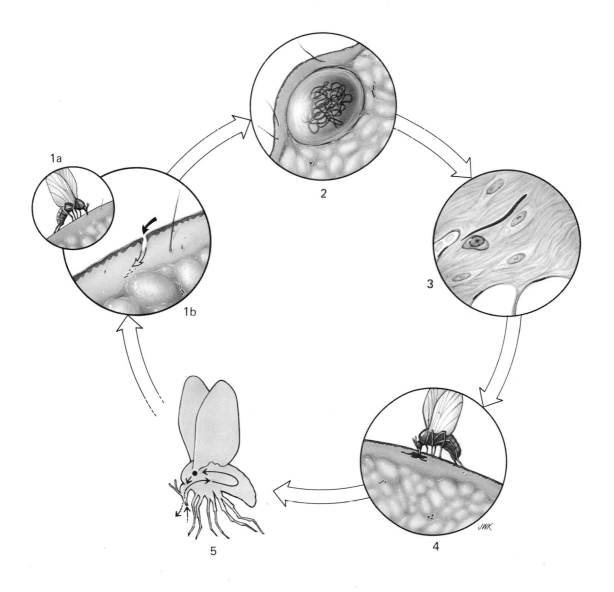

1a

1b

2

3

4

5

*JWK*

Kingdom: Animal
Phylum: Nematoda
Class: Phasmida
Order: Filariata
Family: Onchocercidae
Genus: *Onchocerca*
Species: *volvulus*

# Selected Readings

## General

Ash L, Oriel T: Atlas of Human Parasitology. Chicago, American Society of Clinical Pathologists, 1987

Ash L, Oriel T: Parasites: A Guide to Laboratory Procedures and Identification. Chicago, American Society of Clinical Pathologists, 1987

August JT (ed): Molecular Parasitology. New York and London, Academic Press, 1984

Bailey WS (ed): Cues That Influence Behavior of Internal Parasites. New Orleans, Agricultural Research Service, USDA, 1982

Campbell WC, Rew R (eds): Chemotherapy of Parasitic Diseases. New York and London, Plenum, 1986

Cox FEG (ed): Modern Parasitology. Oxford and London, Blackwell Scientific Publications, 1982

Evered D, Collins GM (eds): Cytopathology of Parasitic Diseases. London, Pitman, 1983

Howell MJ (ed): Parasitology—Quo Vadit. Canberra, Australian Academy of Science, 1986

Katz M, Despommier DD, Gwadz R: Parasitic Diseases. New York and Heidelberg, Springer-Verlag, 1982

Kennedy CR (ed): Ecological Aspects of Parasitology. Amsterdam and Oxford, North-Holland Publishing, 1976

Newton BN, Michal F (eds): New Approaches to the Identification of Parasites and Their Vectors. Basel, Schwabe, 1984

Nicoli RM, Penaud A (eds): 50 Cycles Epidemiologique. Paris, Médicine et Sciences Internationale, 1983

Price PW (ed): Evolutionary Biology of Parasites. Princeton NJ, Princeton University Press, 1980

Rogers WP (ed): The Nature of Parasitism. New York and London, Academic Press, 1962

Peters W, Gilles HM: Color Atlas of Tropical Medicine and Parasitology. Chicago IL, Year Book Medical Publishers, 1977

Schmidt G, Roberts L (eds): Foundations of Parasitology. St. Louis MO, Mosby, 1981

Strickland GT (ed): Hunters' Tropical Medicine. Philadelphia and London, Saunders, 1984

Trager W (ed): Living Together: The Biology of Animal Parasitism. New York, Plenum, 1986

Wakelin D (ed): Immunity to Parasites: How Animals Control Parasite Infections. London, Edward Arnold, 1984

Warren KS, Bowers JZ (eds): Parasitology: A Global Perspective. New York, Springer-Verlag, 1983

Whitfield PJ (ed): The Biology of Parasitism. Baltimore, University Park Press, 1979

## Protozoa

Baker JR: The Biology of Parasitic Protozoa. London, Edward Arnold, 1982

Bruce-Chwatt LJ: Essentials of Malariology. New York, Wiley, 1985

Erlandsen SL, Myer EA (eds): Giardia and Giardiasis. New York, Plenum, 1984

Hudson L (ed): The biology of trypanosomes. Curr Topics Microbioal Immunol 117:183, 1985

Jensen JB (ed): In Vitro Cultivation of Protozoan Parasites. Boca Raton FL, CRC Press, 1983

Lee JJ, Hunter SH, Bovee EC (eds): An Illustrated Guide to the Protozoa. Lawrence KS, Allen Press, 1985

Levine ND, et al: A newly revised classification of the Protozoa. J Protozool, 27:37–58, 1980

Martinez-Paloma A: The Biology of Entamoeba histolytica. Chichester, England, Wiley, 1982

Molyneux DH, Ashford RW (eds): The Biology of Trypanosomes and Leishmania Parasites of Man and Animals. New York, Taylor and Francis, 1983

## Cestodes

Arai MP (ed): Biology of the Tapeworm Hymenolepis Diminuta. New York and London, Academic Press, 1983

Arme C, Pappas PW (eds): Biology of the Eucestoda, Vol 1, 2. New York and London, Academic Press, 1983

Flisser A, Williams K, Laclette C, et al (eds): Cysticercosis: Present State of Knowledge and Perspectives. New York and London, Academic Press, 1982

Schmidt G: Key to the Identification of Tapeworms. Boca Raton, FL, CRC Press, 1986

Thompson RSA, Allen G: Biology of Echinococcus and Hydatid Disease. London, Allen and Unwin, 1986

## Trematodes

Bruce JJ, Sornmani S (eds): The Mekong Schistosome. Whitmore Lake MI, Malacological Review, 1980

Jordan P: Schistosomiasis. The St. Lucia Project. Cambridge, England, Cambridge University Press, 1985

Smyth JD, Halton DW (eds): The Physiology of Trematodes. Cambridge, England, Cambridge University Press, 1983

## Nematodes

Campbell WC (ed): Trichinella and Trichinosis. New York, Plenum, 1983

Croll NA (ed): The Organization of Nematodes. London and New York, Academic Press, 1976

Crompton DWI, Nesheim MC, Pawlowski ZF (eds): Ascariasis and Its Public Health Significance. London and Philadelphia, Taylor and Francis, 1985

Kim CW (ed): Trichinellosis. Albany NY, New York State University Press, 1985

Zuckerman BM (ed): Nematodes as Biological Models, Vol 1, 2. London and New York, Academic Press, 1980

# Alphabetical Listing of Parasites